Illustrated MINAMATA DISEASE

Foundation
Minamata Disease Centre Soshisha
Minamata Disease Museum

Illustrated Minamata Disease
Contents

Foreword 7

1 THE SHIRANUI SEA—a beautiful sea and a bountiful life

THE SHIRANUI SEA is a small and calm sea 11

The sea and the people 12

"EBISU-SAN" (THE DEITY OF WEALTH) near MINAMATA 13

UTASEAMI (TRAWLNET) fishing 14

PURSE SEINE fishing 15

They made everything by themselves in the good old days 16

The local economy depends half on the land and half on the sea 17

Basket used for striped mullet fishing 18

Principal fishing methods in THE SHIRANUI SEA 19

2 MINAMATA DISEASE—CHISSO's crime

CHISSO 23

CHISSO's principal products before THE SECOND WORLD WAR 24

We are surrounded by CHISSO's products 25

CHISSO factory complex at HUNGNAM, KOREA 26

CHISSO factory complex at MINAMATA 27

CHSSO's criminal dumping of mercury into the sea 28

Mercury was used to produce acetaldehyde 29

Methyl mercury drains out of CHISSO into the sea 30

Marine habitats have been lost 31

CHISSO lords it over MINAMATA 32

Mercury travels from fish and shellfish to man 33

Health damage 34

Mercury damages—the nervous cells 35

Mercury passes from mother to fetus 36

MINAMATA disease as a general disorder 37

Dysgraphia 38

A wide range of disabilities for daily life 39

The entire SHIRANUI area was found polluted 40

Application for official certification came from the entire district on the
      SHIRANUI SEA 41

More than 200,000 victims of mercury poisoning 43

More than physical health has been damaged 44

The medical care for MINAMATA disease patients 45

The scope and depth of damage and sufferings 46

MINAMATA disease victims condemned by politicians 47

The kind of mud flung at MINAMATA victims by local people 48

3 A LONG STRUGGLE—Thirty years of victimisation and suffering

Search for the cause and source of MINAMATA disease 51

The cats were the first to go mad and die—1954 52

MINAMATA disease was discovered—1956 53

Nothing was done about the contaminated fish—1957 55

Fishermen rose in protest—1959 56

The patients roused to action at last—1959 57

CHISSO's fraudulent contract—1959 58

The patients' campaign swung into high gear 59

The court ruling on MINAMATA disease—part of the reasons for the decision 60

Compensation agreement—1973 61

Compensation awards as they stand now—9 January 1991 62

Direct negotiations with CHISSO president 63

Patients of the independent negotiation faction sit-in 64

Organised support of the victims 65

Patients' struggle against the certification system 66

The certification system 67

Cons outweigh pros in the application for official certification 68

Applications rejected one after another 69

The number of certified patients 70

4 NOW—What should we do and what can we do ?

> The plight of uncertified patients 73
> The patients are getting old 74
> Many more patients outside KUMAMOTO prefecture 75
> Sediments dredged out and the bay filled in 77
> Mercury was in use all over JAPAN 78
> Patients in protest against the imputation of "FAKE PATIENTS" 80
> MINAMATA disease is not over yet 81
> MINAMATA disease centre SOSHISHA 83

Foreword

Illustrated Minamata Disease presents a vivid picture of Minamata Disease in——historical perspective——a picture largely based on the source materials and photographs on display at the Minamata Disease Museum.

Today we have disturbing reports which tell of mercury poisoning in the Amazon basin and of a great variety and volume of toxic micro-pollutants which are burdening and polluting our earth. In this context of global pollution, it may be indisputable that the significant implications of Minamata Disease for all who inhabit this planet are greater and more serious than ever.

Minamata Disease is not war damage or an unavoidable misdeed. It is not a "Kogai" due to technical failure in industrial processes. What is called a "Kogai" (which literally means "harm or damage to the genral public") in Japan may be defined as "a man-made disaster caused by activities of private and public enterprises which assaults local residents." It is generally believed, however, that a "Kogai" is something you cannnot help accepting because it is assumed to be the result of beneficial industrial activities for improving standards of living.

As a matter of fact, Minamata Disease broke out and has spread as a result of the deliberate pursuit of profit by an irresponsible industrial corporation and of the national government's policy of guidance, acquiescence and protection. Neither the Chisso corporation nor the government has had any pretension to concern and consideration for public welfare or environmental conservation.

Perhaps Japan's remarkable post-war recovery and prosperity due to the national policy of high economic growth was backed by the optimistic idea that industrial progress and national wealth would automatically lead to better welfare for the people. Perhaps a majority of Japanese people supported this ideology and the policies based on it because they were suffering from impoverishments and deprivations in the post-war period. Industrial prosperity and sky-rocketing Gross National Product, however, have brought us where we stand now. Japan is polluted and people are suffering from

Minamata Disease.

It is sincerely hoped that this small book will carry an urgent important message from us in Minamata to those people in Asia, Africa and Latin America who, burdened with poverty and deprivations and striving for economic development, may be thinking of following in the steps of Japan.

Our deepest gratitude goes to the Magsaysay Foundation for its geneous support in financing this book. We would also like to thank Prof. Seiji Minamida, Chiba University, for his help in translating the manuscript into English.

1
THE SHIRANUI SEA

A BEAUTIFUL SEA
AND
A BOUNTIFUL LIFE

THE SHIRANUI SEA IS A SMALL AND CALM SEA

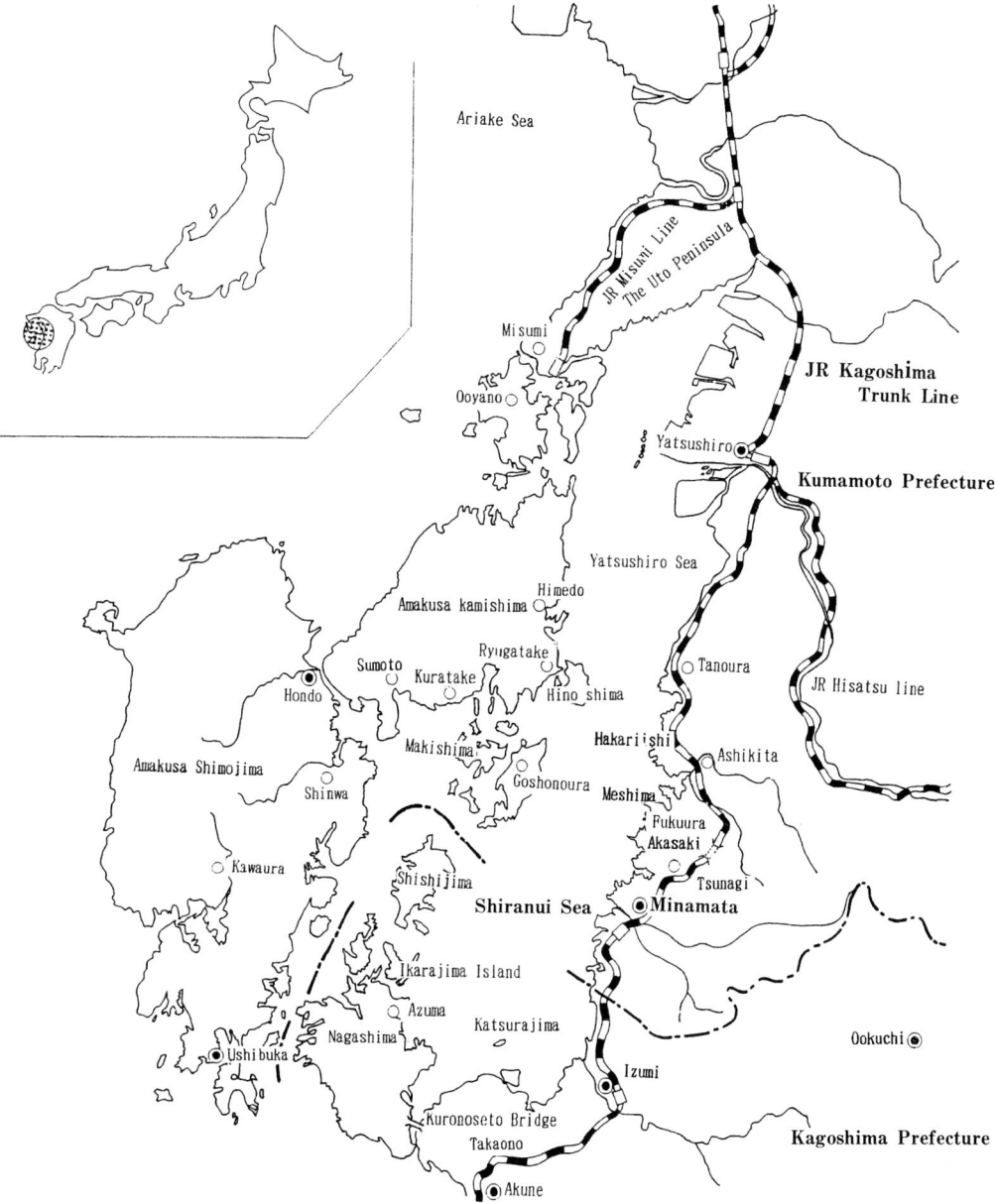

The Shiranui Sea (or the Yatsushiro Sea) is an inland sea surrounded by Kyushu and the Amakusa Islands. It covers an area of nearly 1,400km² (about the size of Lake Biwa), 6 to 16km E. to W., and 70km N. to S.. On average it is about 50m in depth, but the range of ebb and flow is 4m. The coast of the southern part of the Shiranui Sea, where Minamata is located, is ragged with many inlets and coves suitable for the spawning grounds of fish and shellfish. A great variety of creatures live in this area.

THE SEA AND THE PEOPLE

    The Shiranui Sea, as seen from Minamata, reflects in its glassy waters the Amakusa Islands on the opposite side. Except when a typhoon happens to hit this area, fishermen row out to sea in their fishing-boats every day. They celebrate and enjoy their catch of fresh fish with a glass of Shochu (low-class distilled spirits) alone on their boat or at home with their family members. Even villagers from behind an inland range of hills are invited by the briny scent of sea breezes, and come down to the coast to gather oysters or bina (conches). Thus, the Shiranui Sea and the people on the coast have been on friendly terms with each other: the people have been embraced and fostered by the sea that has enabled them to live a simple but happy life blessed with the bounties of nature.

"EBISU-SAN"
(THE DEITY OF WEALTH)
NEAR MINAMATA

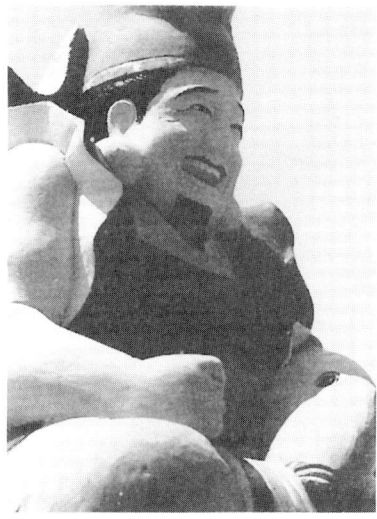

at Umedo Fishing Port

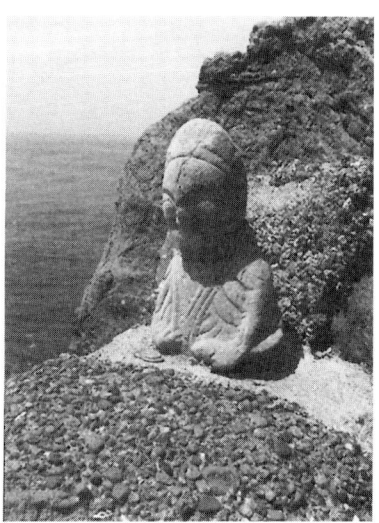

at Umedo Futago Island

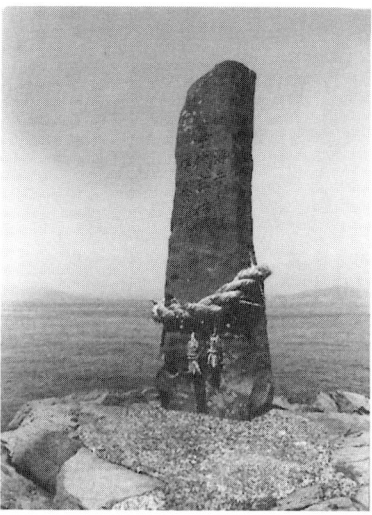

at Umedo Futago Island

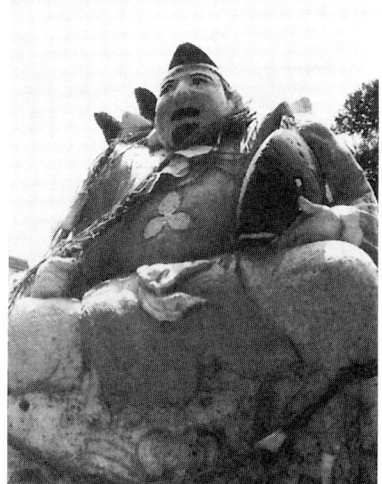

at Marushima Fishing Port

Photographed by Jin Akutagawa 1978

Nearly all fishing villages in this district have stone images of Ebisu ——a Deity who is believed to bring fish to the local fishermen, who used to take a day off, twice a year, to celebrate his blessings. Ebisu images, therefore, indicate the measure of the local fishermen's love and awe for the sea with which they live and thrive.

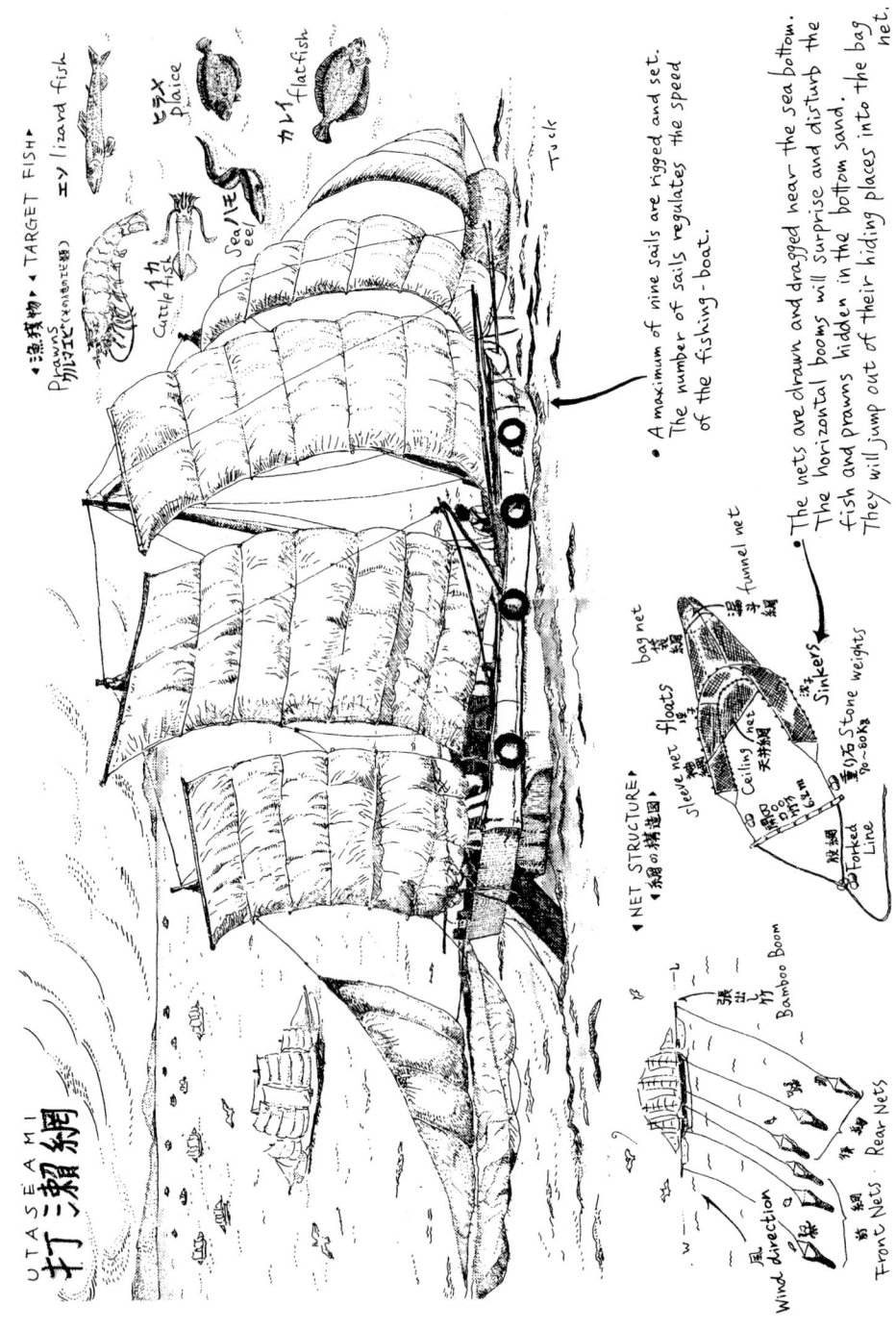

UTASEAMI
(TRAWLNET) FISHING

"Nagare". The trawl-net was not drawn by human power but by that of wind and tide to catch prawns and shrimps, crabs and plaice that live near the sea bottom. This fishing method is rare in Japan.

Drawn by Akemi Takaku 1988

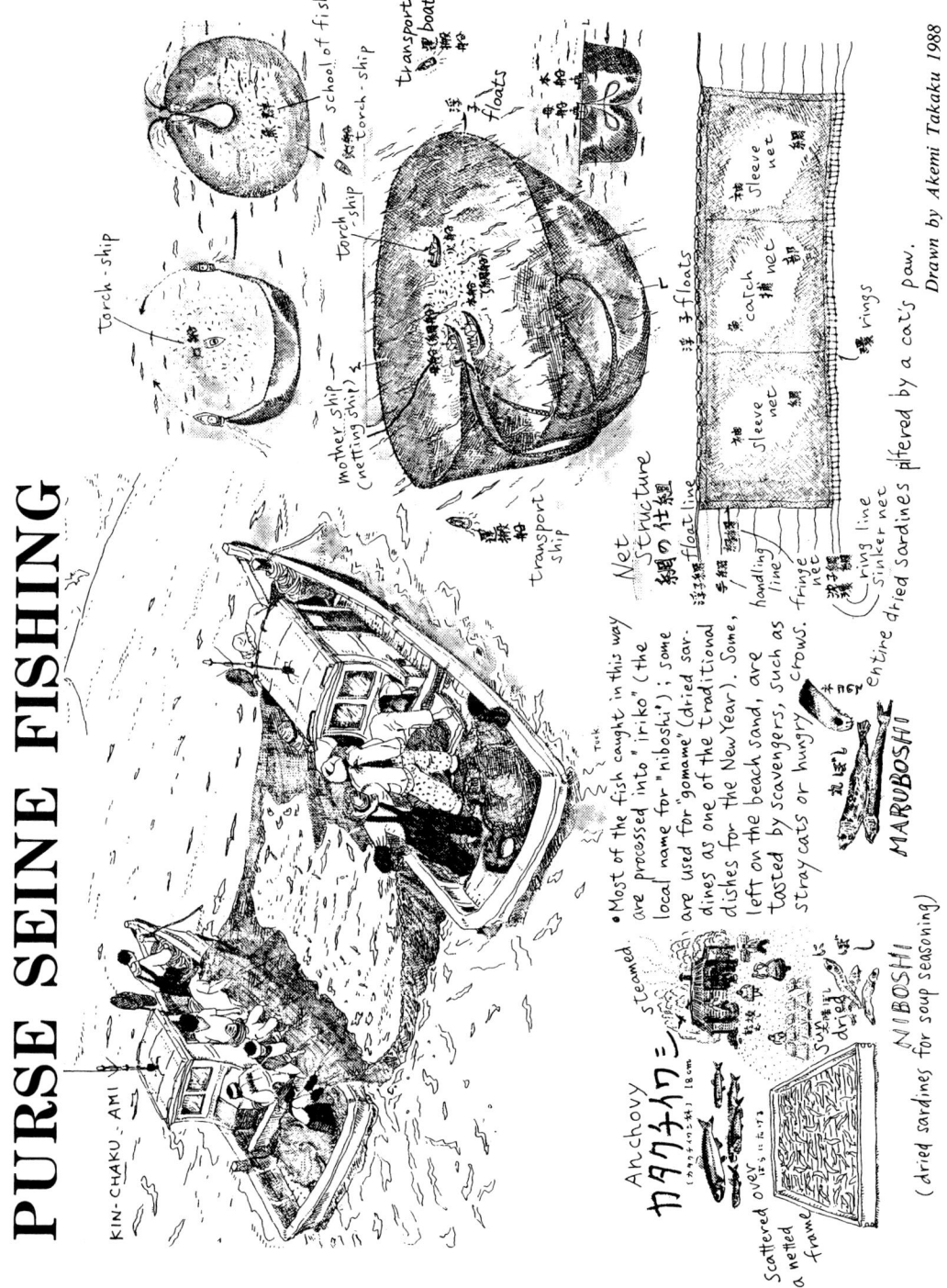

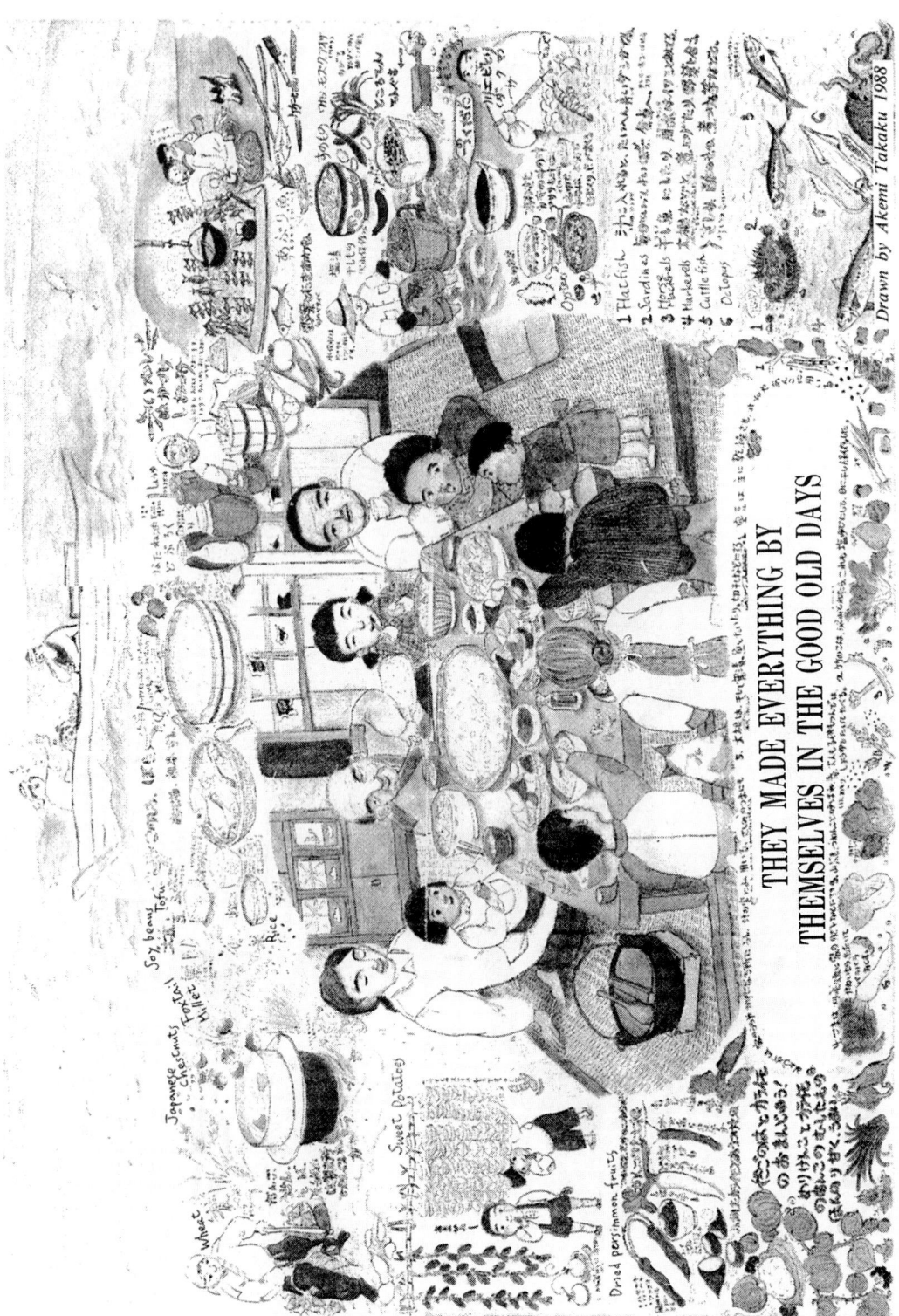

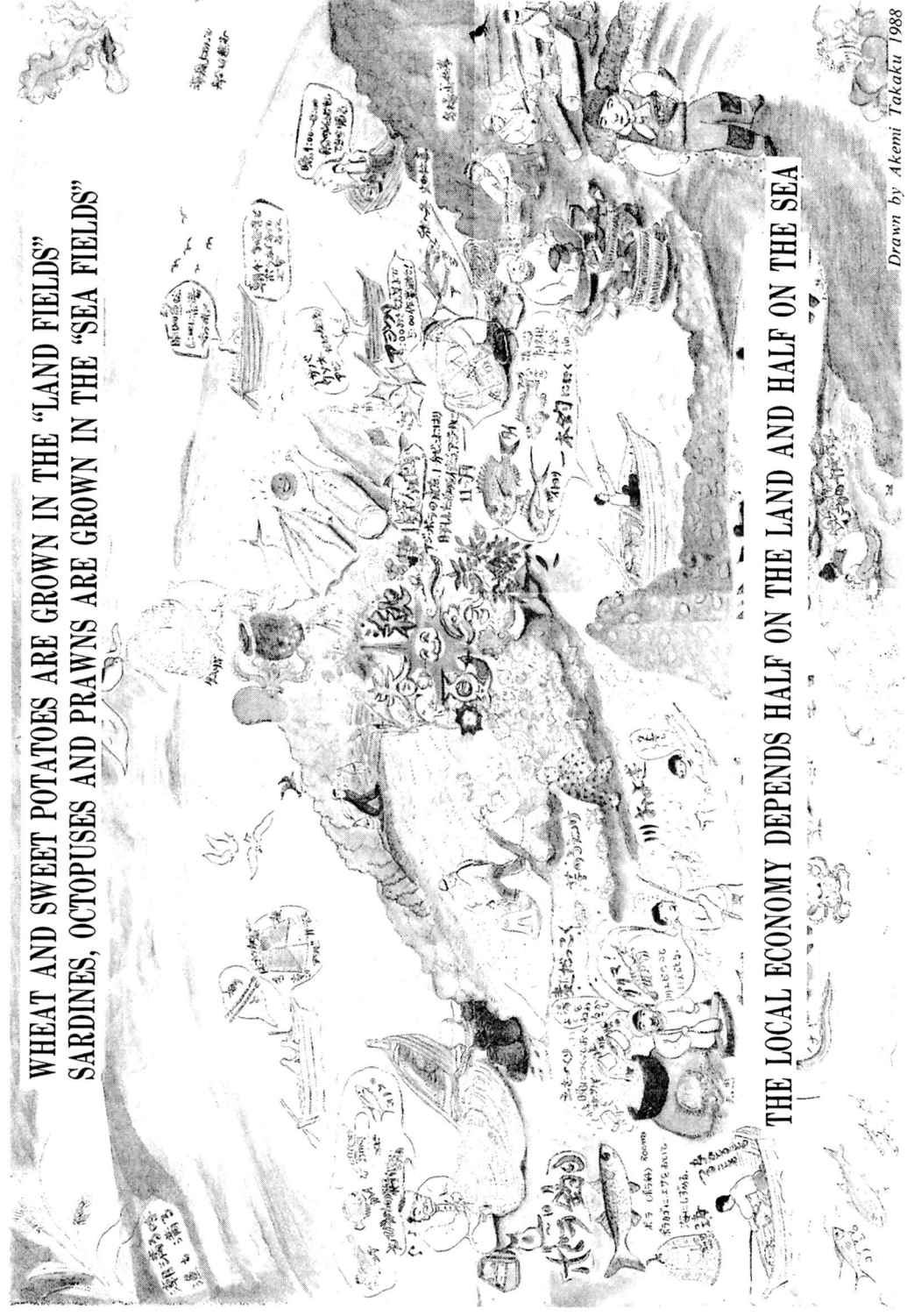

WHEAT AND SWEET POTATOES ARE GROWN IN THE "LAND FIELDS"
SARDINES, OCTOPUSES AND PRAWNS ARE GROWN IN THE "SEA FIELDS"

THE LOCAL ECONOMY DEPENDS HALF ON THE LAND AND HALF ON THE SEA

Drawn by Akemi Takaku 1988

BASKET USED FOR STRIPED MULLET FISHING

Drawn by Akemi Takaku 1988

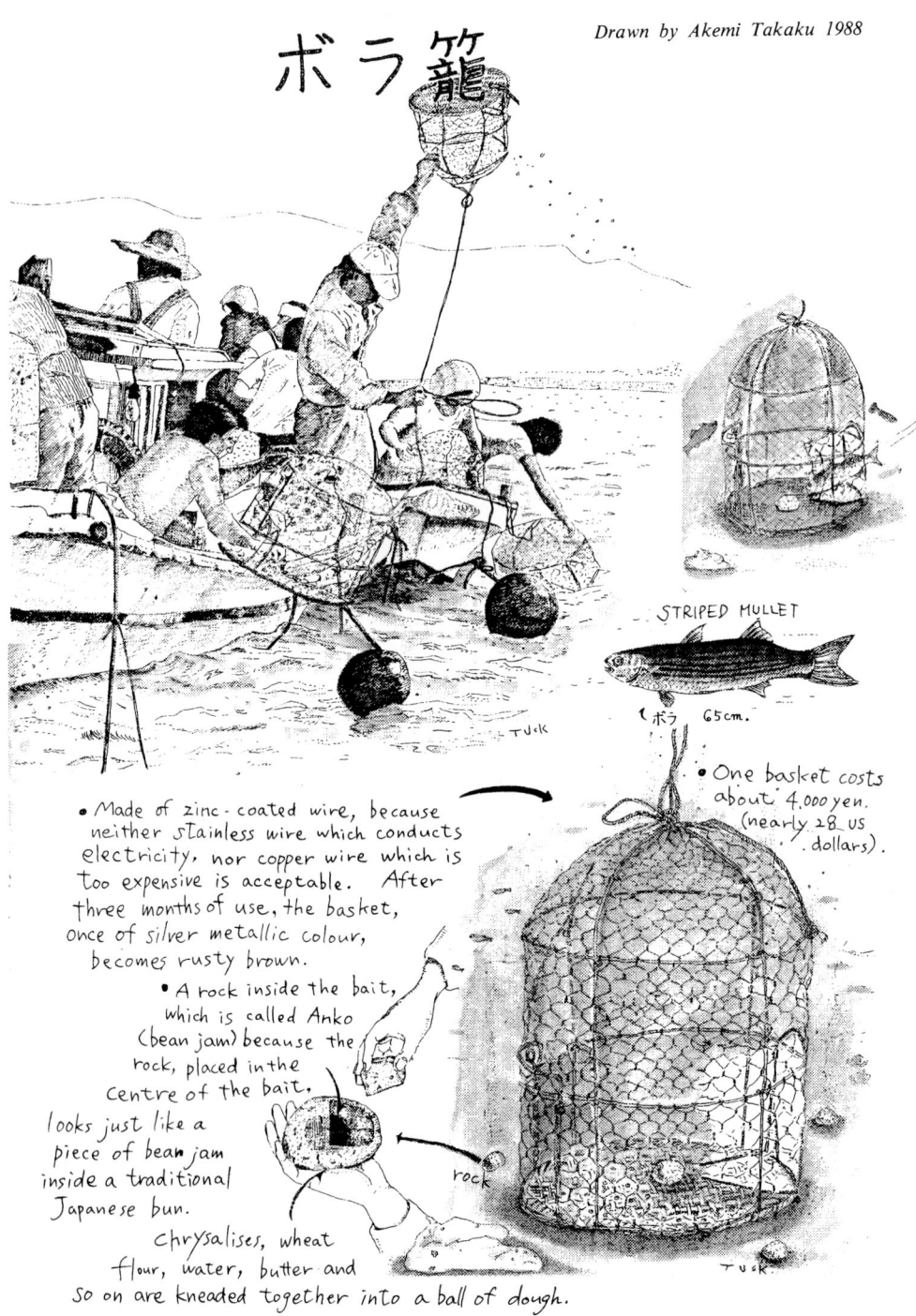

ボラ籠

STRIPED MULLET

ボラ 65cm.

- Made of zinc-coated wire, because neither stainless wire which conducts electricity, nor copper wire which is too expensive is acceptable. After three months of use, the basket, once of silver metallic colour, becomes rusty brown.

- A rock inside the bait, which is called Anko (bean jam) because the rock, placed in the centre of the bait, looks just like a piece of bean jam inside a traditional Japanese bun. Chrysalises, wheat flour, water, butter and so on are kneaded together into a ball of dough.

- One basket costs about 4,000 yen. (nearly 28 US dollars).

rock

PRINCIPAL FISHING METHODS IN THE SHIRANUI SEA

HAND DRAGNET FISHING
This is a variation on the dragnet fishing method carried out in a fishing boat with a small engine. It is used to catch prawns, flatfish, octopuses and cuttlefish in shallow waters. Popular at Taura.

DRAGNET FISHING FOR BAIT
This is also a variation on the dragnet fishing method carried out in a fishing-boat with a small engine. It is used to catch small bait fish to be used as bait for rod fishing and long-line fishing. It is in use now at Goshonoura to catch live shrimps for pole-and-line fishing for sea breams.

DRAGNET FISHING FOR CLAMS
This is also a variation on the dragnet fishing method carried out in a fishing-boat with a small engine.

DRAGNET FISHING FOR TREPANG
This is also a variation on the dragnet fishing method carried out in a fishing-boat with a small engine.

TRAWLNET FISHING
This is a variation on the trawlnet fishing method carried out in a small fishing-boat. You stop your engine, cast your net and let your boat drift with the wind. It is mainly employed at Hakariishi, Ashikita County, to catch Ishiebi (Stone Shrimps), prawns, cuttlefish, sea eels, Eso and plaice.

PURSE SEINE FISHING
This is a variation on the round haul net fishing carried out in a medium-sized fishing-boat. It is mainly used to catch anchovies, as well as to catch sardines, horse mackerels and mackerels. Most sardines are made into "iriko" (soup seasoning) but some of them are used as live bait for bonito fishing. This method is restricted to Shishi Island and to the east coast of Amakusa.

IMPROVED NET FISHING
This is a variation on the round haul net fishing carried out in a small fishing-boat. This one is smaller than a purse seine net but an improved version of it. It is used to catch sardines for "iriko" and anchovies as well.

GOCHI AMI FISHING
This is similar to the hand dragnet fishing method in that a small number of fishermen handle their net, but different in that the net is just dropped, not drawn by the boat. It is the most typical method employed in the Shiranui Sea to catch sea breams, guchi, sea eels and cutlass fish.

POLE-AND-LINE FISHING
This method is used to catch sea breams, horse mackerels, octopuses, grunts and blow-fish. Tackles and techniques depend on which season of the year you work in, what kind of fish you look for and where.

SPEAR FISHING
This is usually done at night. You thrust your spear at the head of your fish.

OCTOPUS FISHING
You wade at hip-depth in the sea and look for your octopus with a glass-bottomed box held in one hand. When you find one, you thrust your spear at it.

POWER-DRAWN TRAWLNET FISHING FOR SARDINES
This is used to catch anchovies to be made into "iriko".

GILL NET FISHING
This is an old traditional fishing method. One to three nets are cast across the direction of the current to entangle fish by the gills. It is used to catch prawns, crabs and Kutsusoko.

BASKET FISHING FOR CUTTLEFISH
Baskets are dropped to the sea bottom to catch pregnant cuttlefish swarming inshore to spawn.

BASKET FISHING FOR STRIPED MULLETS
Baskets with baits inside are laid at the sea bottom to trap them.

BASKET FISHING FOR CRABS
Baskets with baits inside are laid at the sea bottom to trap them.

POT FISHING FOR OCTOPUSES
Pots are dropped to the sea bottom to catch them.

HAZE NET FISHING
This is a variation on the fixed shore net fishing method and a unique fishing method employed in shallow waters off Yatsushiro. A row of bamboo cuttings are placed around the opening of the net to lead fish inside, such as flathead, prawns and flatfish.

FIXED SHORE NET FISHING
This used to be one of the most typical fishing methods employed in the Shiranui Sea until the late 1920s. It was mainly used to catch anchovies. The net was drawn ashore by the whole village.

LONG LINE FISHING
The most typical line is the one with dozens of hooks on it to catch Garakabu (scorpion fish).

OYSTER GATHERING
A special hand tool is used to break oyster shells clinging to the rocks and take the meat out.

BINA CONCH GATHERING
Conches are gathered at ebb tide.

The Shiranui Sea provides spawning grounds for a great variety of fish, which in turn has enabled the early development of diverse fishing methods with rods, nets, pots or baskets. The most typical fish is sardines that used to be caught with fixed shore nets until the introduction of power fishing boats. Then round haul nets (i.e. purse seine nets) came into use. This ishing method required a lot of manpower and funding, which brought into being the division of master fishermen and employed fishermen. In the late 1950s and the early 1960s, many master fishermen found themselves financially in deep waters owing to a sharp decline in the catch of sardines, the introduction of a new wage system and the outbreak of Minamata Disease. Thus, large-scale fishing was abandoned and replaced by small-scale fishing with the use of Gochi nets or gill nets. Moreover, in the mid-60s, fish culture was introduced into the Shiranui Sea area and an increasing number of fishermen have since converted, so that artificially raised fish and shellfish account for more than half of the fish sales in this area now. Hence the serious nature of the mercury contamination of coastal waters.

2
MINAMATA DISEASE
CHISSO'S CRIME

CHISSO

Chisso is descended from the Sogi Electric Company, founded in 1906 at Oguchi village, Kagoshima. In 1908 they started manufacturing chemical fertilisers, which made their fortune. After the First World War, they took another step forward and built another plant in Korea in 1927. Their success in Korean Peninsula enabled them to become one of the biggest chemical manufacturers in Japan.

Chisso had its headquarters and main factory complex in Minamata where they ruled the roost like a feudal lord over his domain. Minamata was under the umbrella of Chisso's economic and social supremacy.

The key to their rapid rise in power and influence was its policy of "Profit first and safety last". Chisso had to catch up with the old giant "Zaibatsus" or concerns who had an earlier start.

CHISSO'S PRINCIPAL PRODUCTS BEFORE THE SECOND WORLD WAR

Fertilisers: Ammonium Sulphate   Ammonium Sulphate Phosphate   Ammonium Sulfide Phosphate   Lime Nitrogen   Superphosphate of Lime   Synthetic Fertiliser

Artificial Silks (Synthetic Fibres):
Bemberg Silk Fibre   Viscose Fibre   Staple Fibre   Rayon Acetate

Explosives: Colloid Dynamite   Ammonium Nitrate Dynamite   Ammonium Nitrate Explosive Black Mining Explosive   Fuse Powder   Slow-burning Fuse Industrial Detonator Electric Detonator Detonator Scissors

Oils: Hardened Oil   Glycerol   Fattyy Acid   Sterol   Pressed Stearin Margarine   Stearic Acid for Rubber   Fatty Acid for Soap   Soap   Dark Oil Soybean Oil

Industrial Chemicals: Aqueous Ammonia Anhydrous Ammonia Liquid Ammonia 40% Nitric Acid 98% Nitric Acid   Ammonium Nitrate Glacial Acetic Acid   Acetic Anhydride Acetone Carbide Minalit Minaloid Vinyl Acetate Chissoloid Sulphuric Acid   Hydrochloric Acid Liquid Chloride   Bleaching Powder Copper Sulphate
Caustic Soda   Soda Ash   Ammonium Chloride Sodium Nitrite Sodium Fluorosilicate Sodium Silicate Formic Acid Oxlic Acid Pentaerythritol   Anhydrous Aluminium Chloride Ethylene Glycol Asahi Aji (synthetic seasoning)   Amino Acid Sauce   Starch

Coal Chemistry: Coal   Heavy Oil   Volatile Oil   Brisquette   Semi-coke Asphalt Pitch Paraffin   Creosote   Koda   Methanol   Formalin   Hexamethylene Tetramine Axel Oil   Synthetic Tannin Chissolite Plywood   Chisolite Compound   Chissolite Plastic

Miscellaneous: Oxygen   Nitrogen   Argon Carbon Electrode   Carbon Black Mercury Magnesium Clinker   Magnesium Metal   Magnesium Alloy Pig Iron Synthetic Jewels

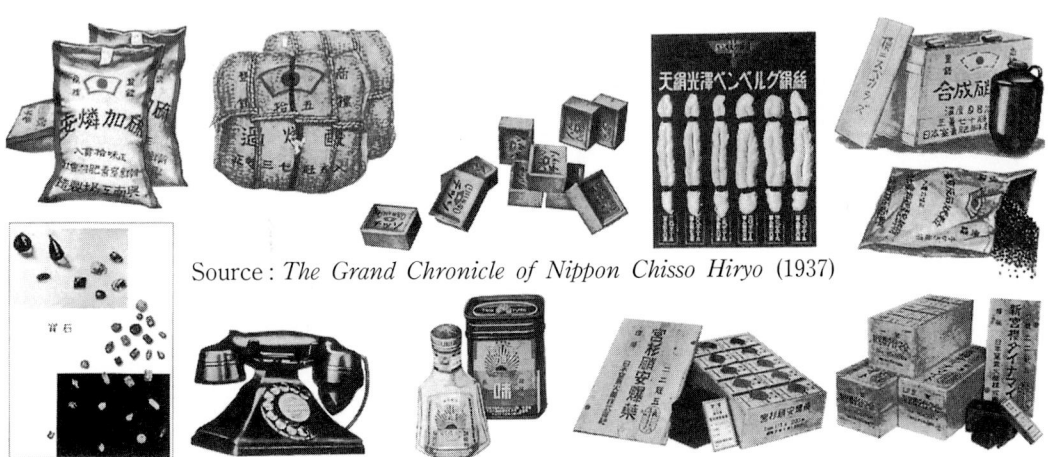

Source: *The Grand Chronicle of Nippon Chisso Hiryo* (1937)

Chisso, as a "general manufacturer of chemicals", used to produce a great variety of chemicals, ranging from daily necessaries such as soaps and synthetic seasonings, through industrial chemicals such as acetic acid and sulphuric acid, to products for military purposes such as explosives. Thus, it was asserted that "Chisso's growth and prosperity reflects the history of the chemical industry as a whole in Japan". Chisso used to enjoy the world-wide reputation of the pioneer and leader of Japanese industry.

WE ARE SURROUNDED BY CHISSO'S PRODUCTS

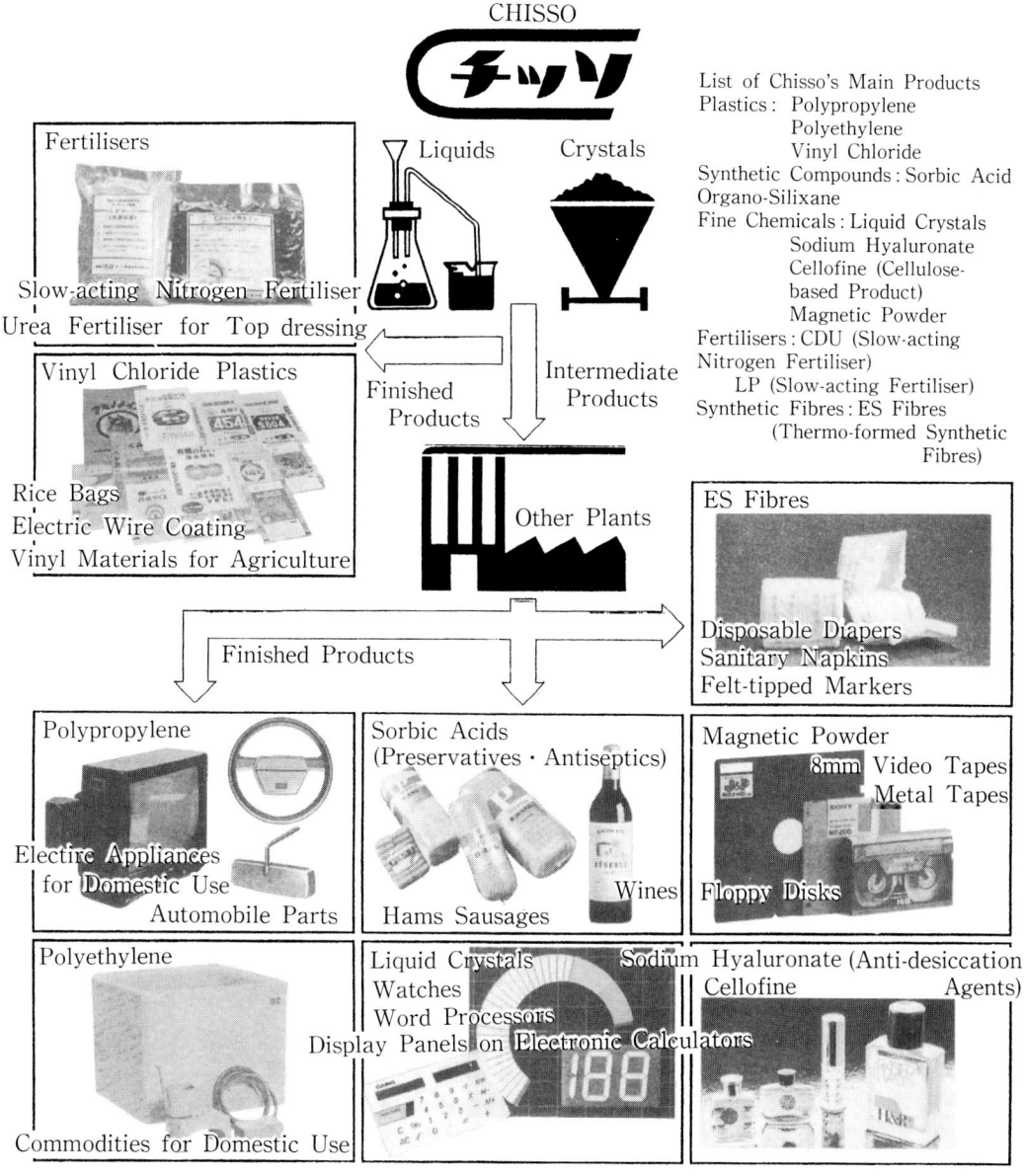

Chisso produces a great variety of finished products and intermediate products, whose presence in our daily life is quite conspicuous. Chisso's technology has, in a way, contributed to the improved conveniences and amenities of our life. In fact, Japan's economic growth and prosperity is mostly due to that of the chemical industry with Chisso as one of its leaders. But the price we have to pay for it is Minamata Disease.

CHISSO FACTORY COMPLEX AT HUNGNAM, KOREA

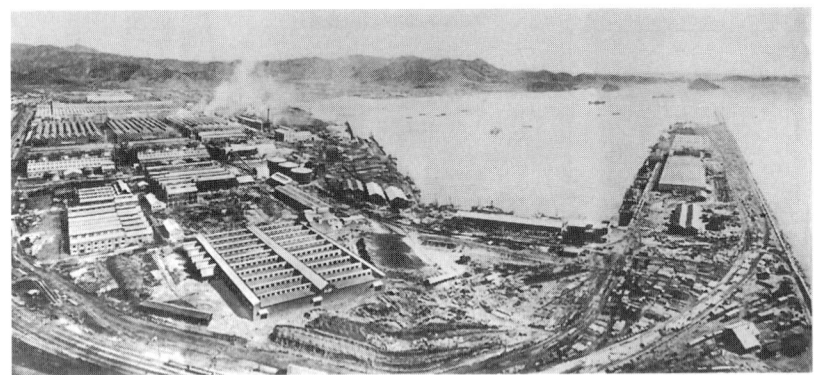

By the latter half of the 1920s, Chisso had accumulated a large amount of profit by manufacturing and selling ammonia sulphate. In 1927 they decided to build another plant at Hungnam in the north of Korea. Hungnam was a small village with a population of about 3,000 inhabitants who lived by fishing and farming. In a few years, the village was transformed beyond recognition. With the Japanese Imperial Army at their back, Chisso succeeded in constructing an enormous complex of factory buildings. In addition, they employed their large financial resources to construct one huge dam after another for electricity supply, a railway line, a hospital and a housing estate for their employees. The Imperial Army helped in evacuating the local inhabitants and there came into being the largest Japanese colony in Asia (with a population of 200,000 in its heyday). The Korean workers they employed were deliberately subjected to severe drudgery: they were dubbed "bulls and horses at the plough".

Source: *The Grand Chronicle of Nippon Chisso Hiryo*

CHISSO FACTORY COMPLEX AT MINAMATA

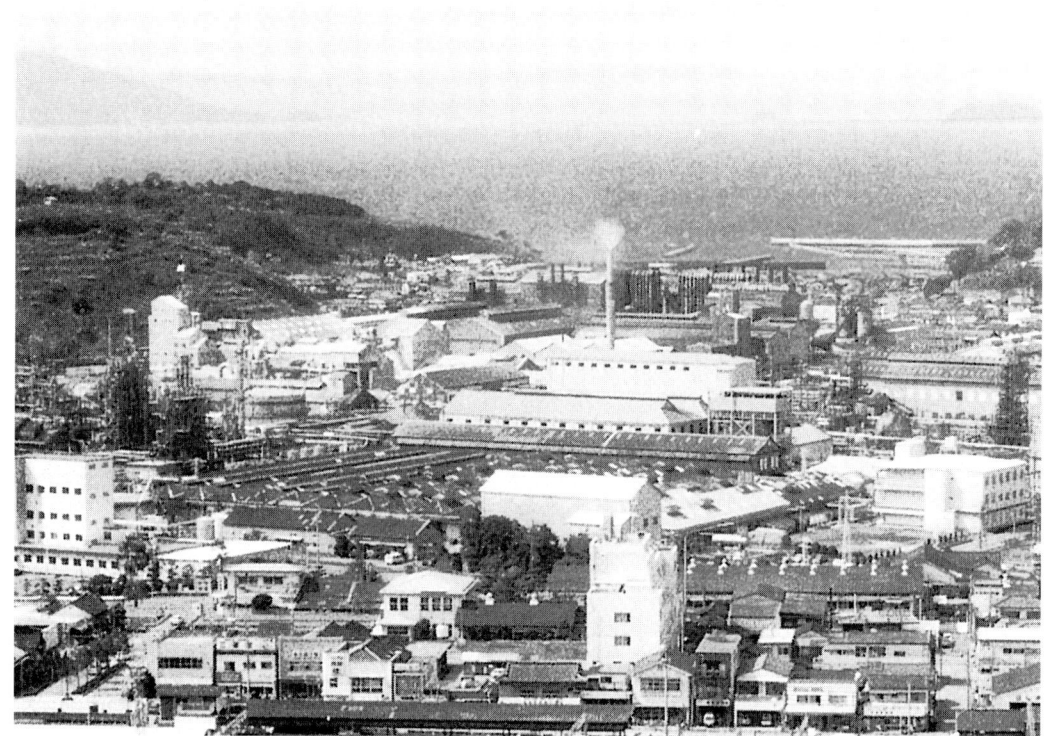

Photographed by Iwao Onizuka 1988

   Still located in the centre of Minamata City, the factory is very old and falling into decay now. There remain some signs of its old prosperity, but only one-fifth of the facilities in its vast premises are in operation today.

CHISSO'S CRIMINAL DUMPING OF MERCURY INTO THE SEA

It is quite evident that Minamata Disease was caused by the effluents that Chisso discharged, untreated, into Minamata Bay. They contained methyl mercury used as a catalyst in manufacturing acetaldehyde. The mercury-contaminated effluents were released for as long as 36 years, starting in 1932. In 1959, these toxic discharges were identified as the cause of Minamata Disease, but Chisso continued to dump mercury into the Bay for nine more years. A large accumulation of toxic substances, including mercury, is found, even today, in the slimy sludge at the bottom of Minamata Bay and it is even spreading all over the Shiranui Sea.

MERCURY WAS USED TO PRODUCE ACETALDEHYDE

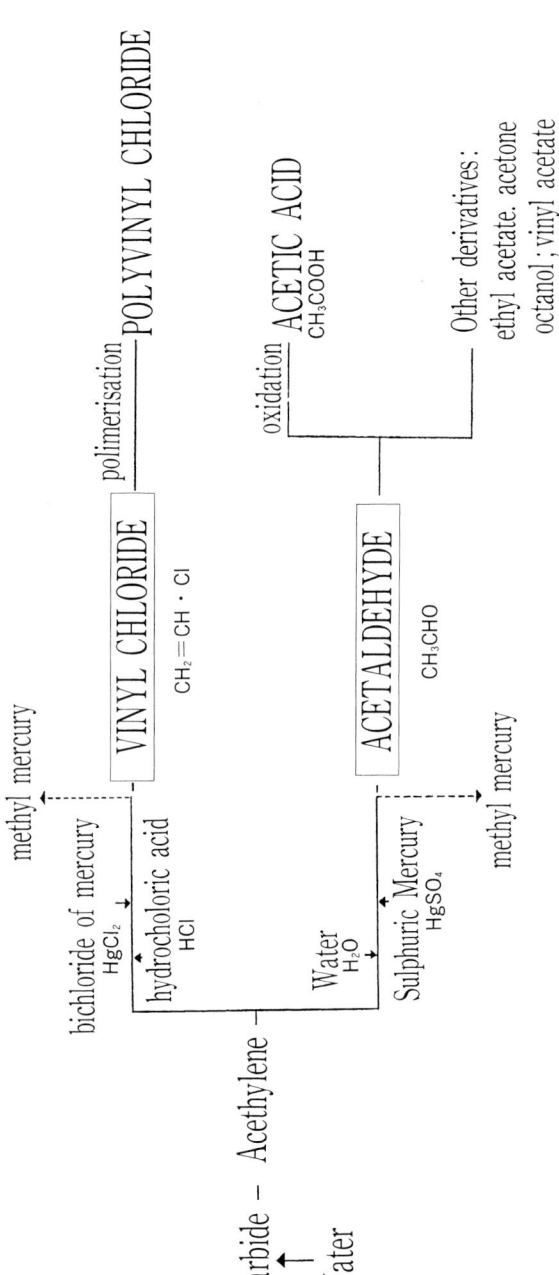

Sulphuric mercury was used at Chisso, Minamata, as a catalyst in produing acetalydehyde, the material for synthetic acetic acid. In this process, the inorganic sulphuric mercury became organic; that is, methyl mercury was produced. Mercury is well-known for its high toxicity, but when it is methylated, its ability to combine with protein is enhanced and thus its toxicity is highly increased. Methyl mercury smells like a rotten egg as it evaporates directly from its crystals.

METHYL MERCURY DRAINS OUT OF CHISSO INTO THE SEA

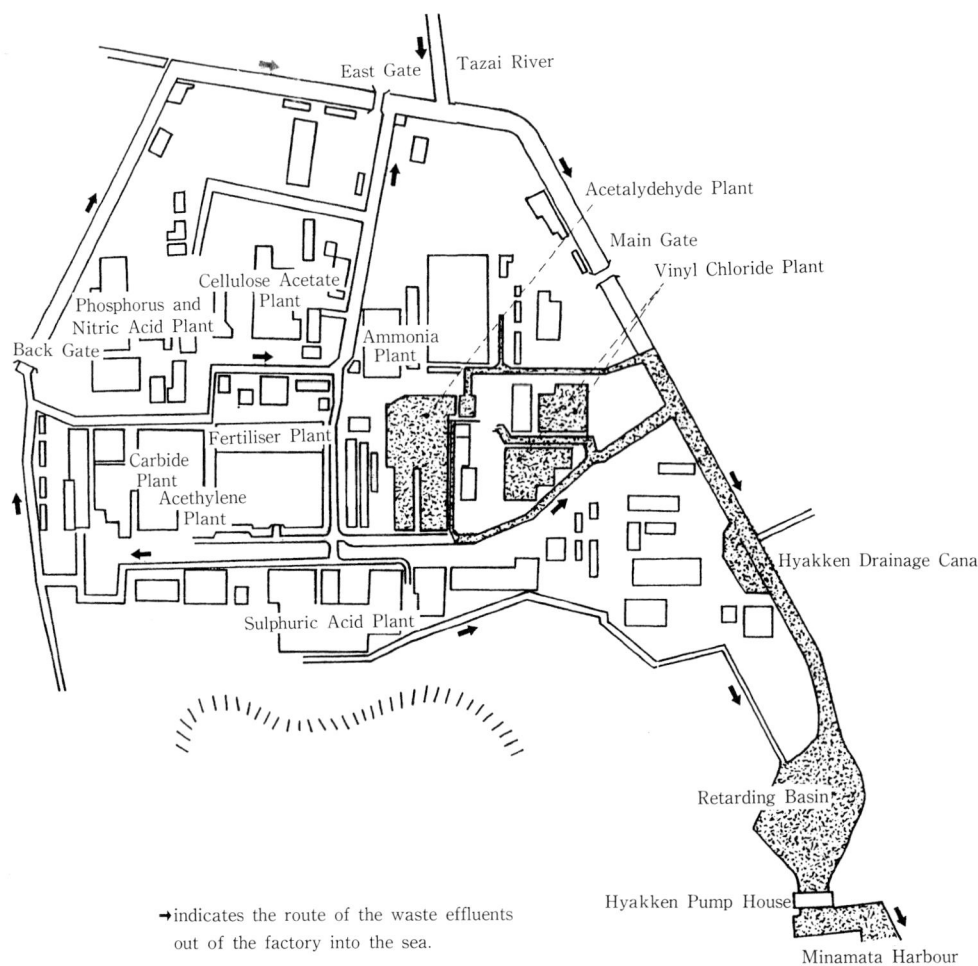

→ indicates the route of the waste effluents out of the factory into the sea.

    Chisso's toxic effluents with methyl mercury in them was discharged into the sea, untreated, for 36 years (from 1932 to 1968). (They included other poisonous heavy metals and chemicals, such as selenium, thalium and manganese.) The total amount of methyl mercury released is estimated at 400--600 tons. It is widely believed that all the mercurial sludge at the sea bottom cannot be recovered.

MARINE HABITATS HAVE BEEN LOST

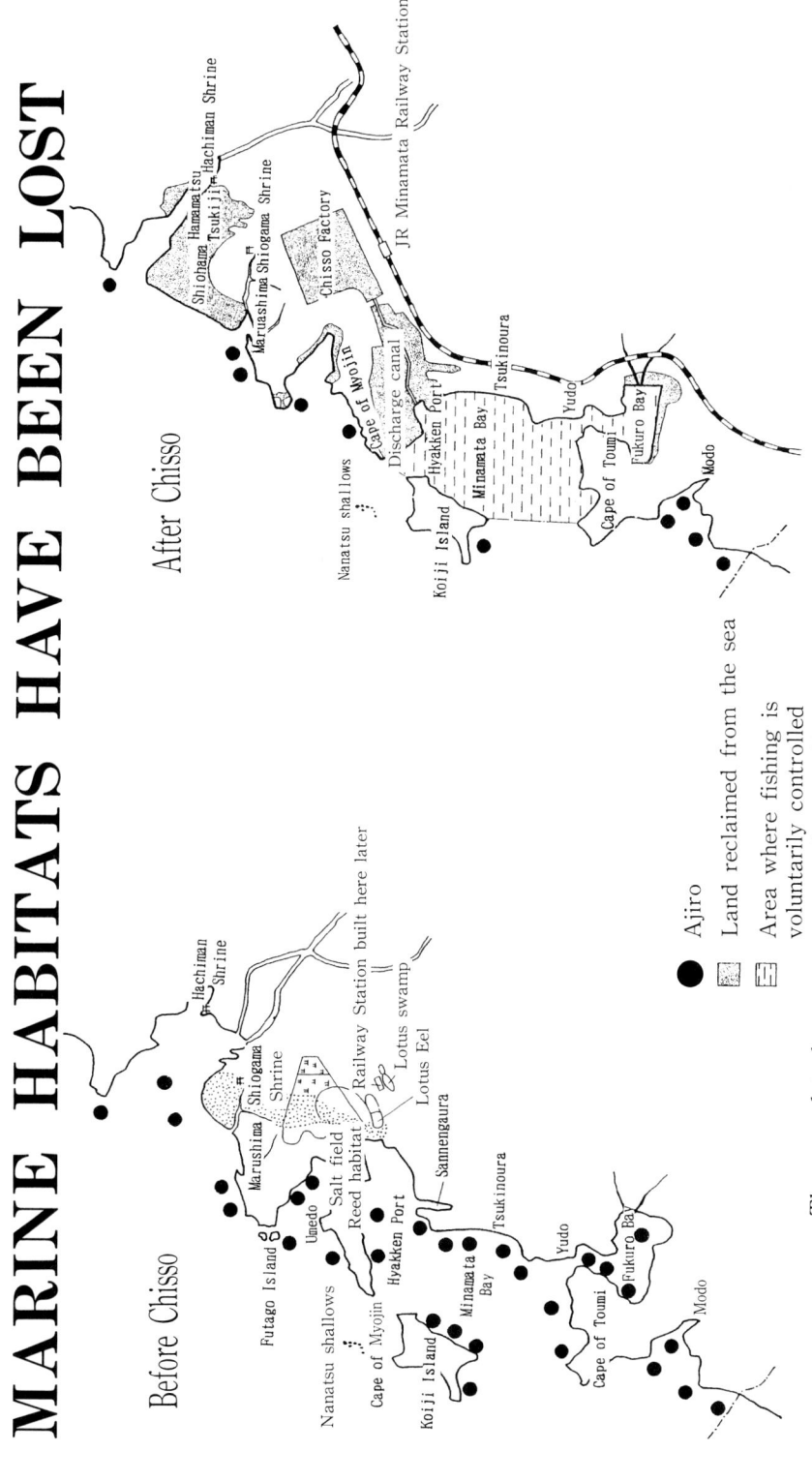

There used to be a great many places, called Ajiro, where many kinds of fishes tended to gather and live, both inside Minamata Bay and near its neighbouring coasts, but most of them have disappeared. Chiss'os effluents settled on the bottom of Minamata Bay. Some fishing ports had to be dredged; other coastal areas had to be drained and filled up; a large discharge pool had to be constructed. That is how most Ajiros were destroyed. Chisso has killed the fertile sea.

CHISSO LORDS IT OVER MINAMATA

- Chisso-owned housing estate for their employees
- Land owned by Chisso (except for housing estates)
- Built-up area
- Agricultural land
- Factory
- Downtown
- Area for public use
- Local council housing estate

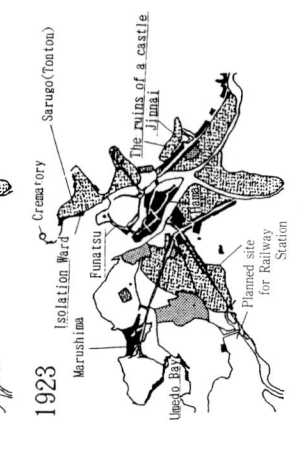

1900

1911

1923
- Sarugo (Tonton)
- Crematory
- The Ruins of a castle
- Jinnai
- Isolation Ward
- Planned site for Railway Station
- Marushima
- Funatsu
- Umedo Bay

- Chisso-related area
- Area for public use
- Built-up area
- Agricultural land
- Salt field
- Local council housing estate

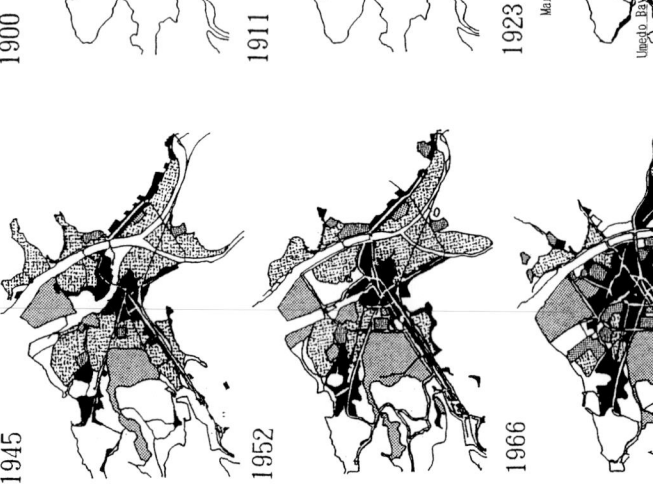

1945

1952

1966

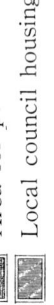

1981

Soon after their arrival at Minamata, Chisso rapidly grew in its power and influence over the political and economic life of Minamata. For example, Mr. Hikoshichi Hashimoto, former director of the Minamata Factory, was elected as Mayor. It was Mr. Hashimoto who invented the method of synthesizing acetic acid which was responsible for Minamata Disease. Another fact in point is the way Chisso acquired more and more land in Minamata as years passed. Chisso sold Hachiman Pool and some other land to the municipal government in the late 1980s, so they own less land now than they did in 1981.

MERCURY TRAVELS FROM FISH AND SHELLFISH TO MAN

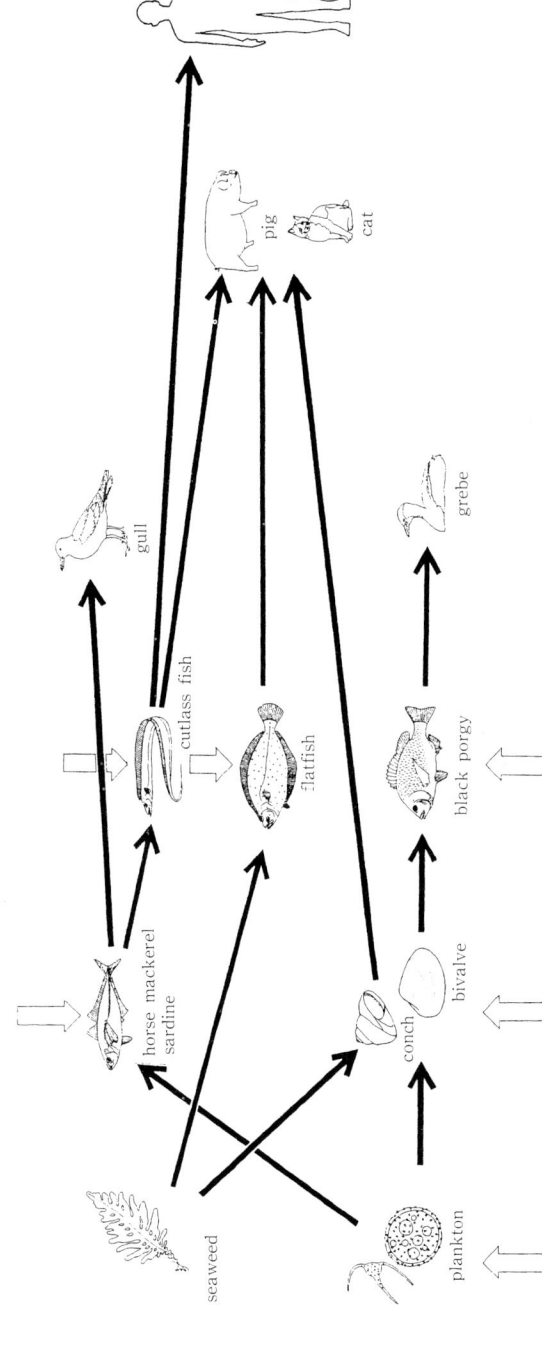

It is true that methyl mercury in the effluents, when discharged into the sea, is diluted, but it is also true that, as it travels through the food chain, it is concentrated tens or hundreds of thousand-fold and accumulates in the internal systems of marine creatures. Methyl mercury is absorbed by plankton that are eaten by fish and shellfish. It is also directly absorbed through fish's gills and skin. Some fish, like striped mullets, take their food with the mud at the seabed, and the mercury sediments in the mud go into their systems. Fish, too, got Minamata Disease. Then came birds, cats, dogs and pigs that ate these fishes. Finally, man became ill. Local inhabitants were horrified and panic-stricken at the "Cat's Dancing Disease" or the "Strange Disease".

HEALTH DAMAGE

Minamata Disease is defined as a disease that you get if an accumulation of methyl mercury in the internal system damages, mainly, your central nervous system as well as your peripheral nerves. Its characteristic symptoms include sensory disturbances, incoordination (ataxia), dysarthsia, disturbance of the visual field, loss of bearings, tremor and many others. In fact, the entire bodily system is affected. The total number of local inhabitants who ate mercury-contaminated fish are estimated at two hundred thousand, so it is quite possible that there may be a lot more latent patients than have come to light. But a full-scale medical investigation of all the local residents, though advocated by many, has never been conducted.

MERCURY DAMAGES THE NERVOUS CELLS

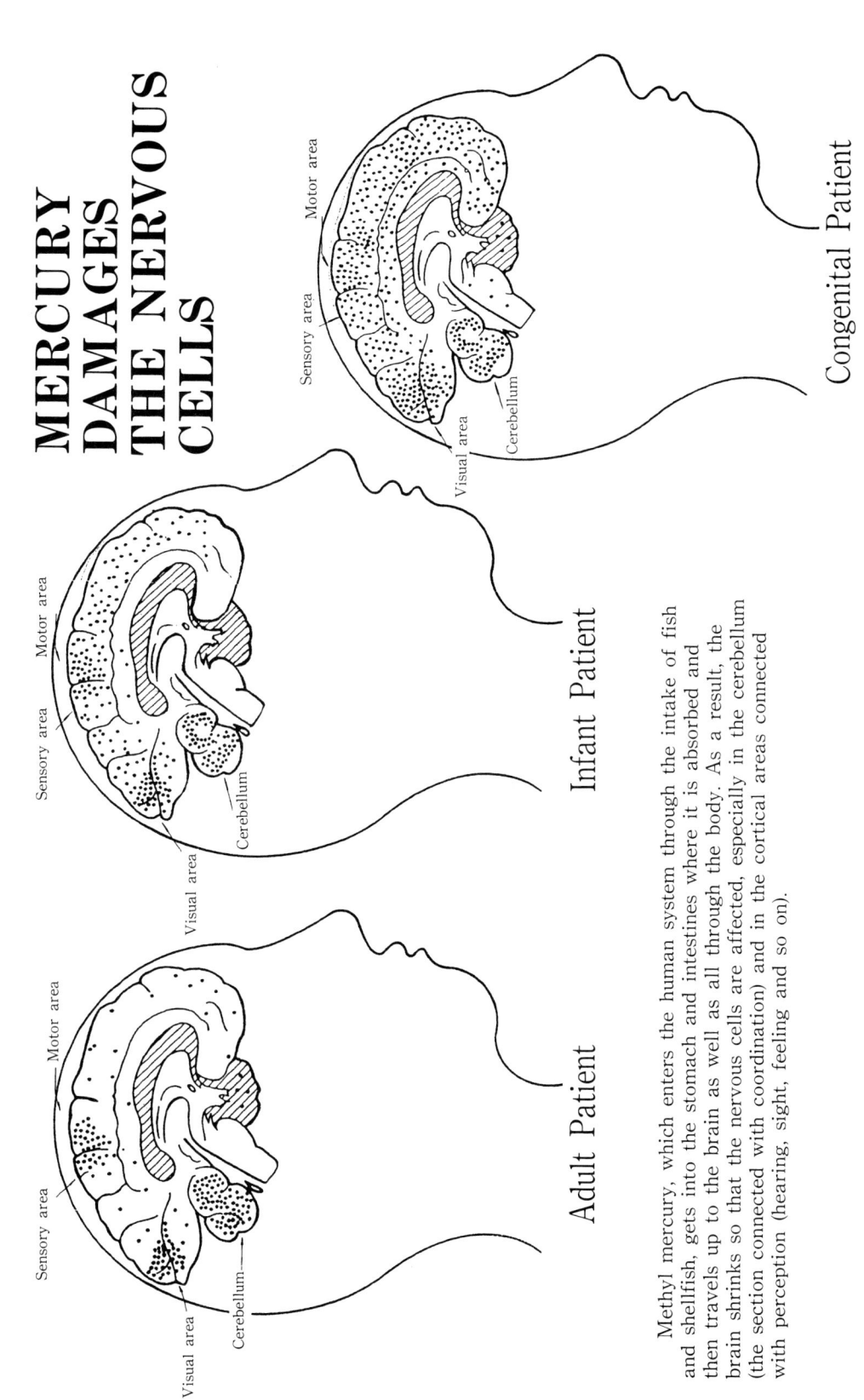

Adult Patient

Infant Patient

Congenital Patient

* Little dots indicate the range and degree of damage caused by methyl mercury in each section.

Methyl mercury, which enters the human system through the intake of fish and shellfish, gets into the stomach and intestines where it is absorbed and then travels up to the brain as well as all through the body. As a result, the brain shrinks so that the nervous cells are affected, especially in the cerebellum (the section connected with coordination) and in the cortical areas connected with perception (hearing, sight, feeling and so on).

MERCURY PASSES FROM MOTHER TO FETUS

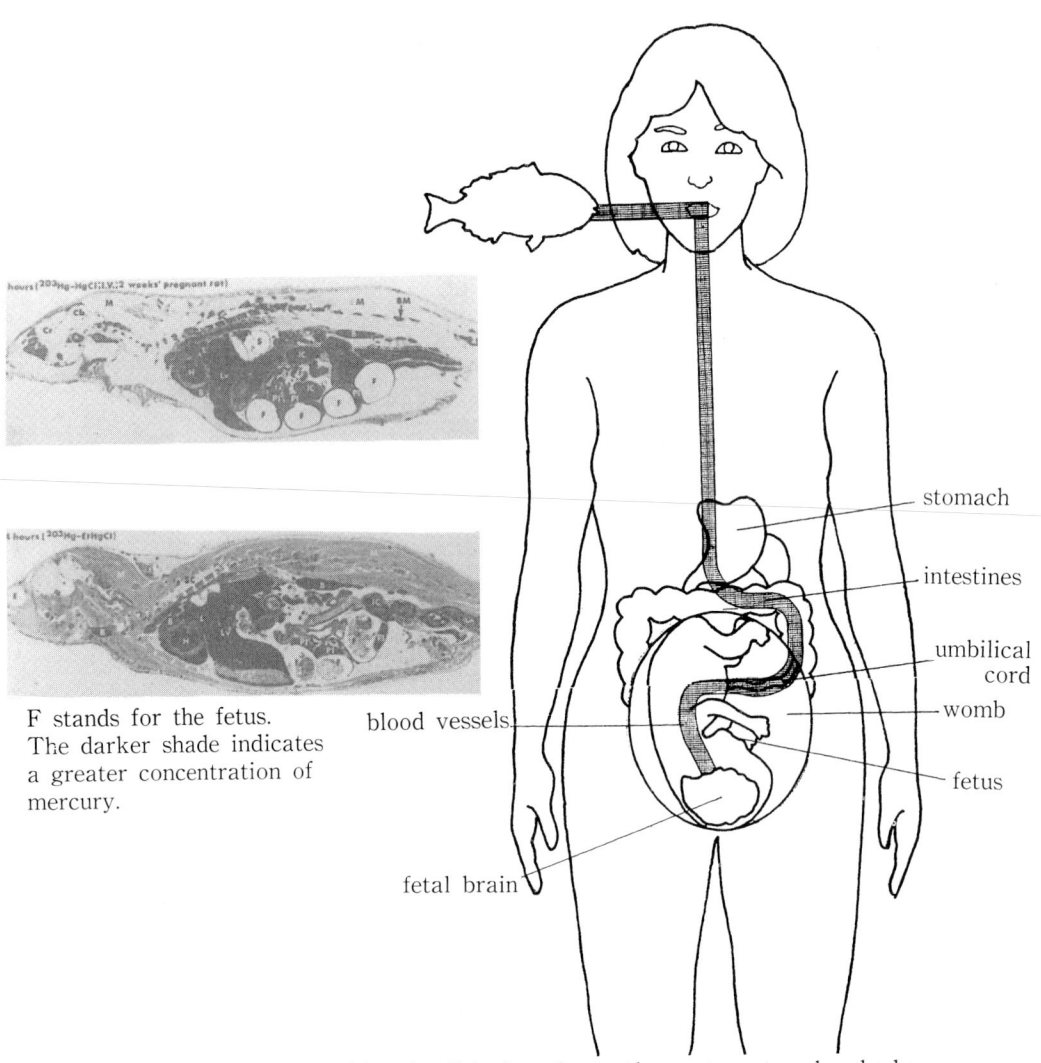

F stands for the fetus. The darker shade indicates a greater concentration of mercury.

Methyl mercury, carried by the fish that the mother eats, enters her body and travels all through it. It also enters the fetus through the umbilical cord. Figure 1 shows a mouse in the second week of pregnancy that had an intravenous injection of inorganic mercury (Hg-HCl : mercury chloride) 24 hours previously. Figure 2 shows a mouse in the same length of pregnancy that had an intravenous injection of organic mercury (Hg-EtHgCl : mercuric ethyl chloride) 24 hours previously. It is quite clear that most of the inorganic mercury is concentrated in the internal organs whereas organic mercury has spread all through the body and even invaded the brain. Organic mercury has also passed through the placenta and affected the fetus.

Source : Hiroji Shiraki

MINAMATA DISEASE AS A GENERAL DISORDER

Researched by Tokichi Rokutanda 1974

Subjective Symptoms

Symptoms	Male(%)	Female(%)
forgetfulness	85.9	83.6
powerlessness	80.4	75.2
ataxicgait	76.4	70.8
numbness of hands and feet	74.8	73.3
difficulty in hand and foot movements	72.4	67.0
tremor of hands and feet	71.5	59.4
disturbances of sight	71.2	78.6
general heaviness	70.6	73.6
pains and heaviness in the head	66.9	70.4
pains in neck, shoulders and sides	64.7	74.2
pains in the hip	63.8	63.2
sleeplessness	62.6	69.8
impaired hearing	62.3	55.3
speech disturbance	61.0	51.3
convulsions	60.7	64.2
vertigo	56.1	62.3
ringing in the ears	51.2	58.5
pains in the joints	47.9	50.6
general numbness	36.8	36.2
general pains	33.7	28.6
general convulsions	29.1	31.4
salivation	28.2	28.9
miscellaneous	5.5	6.6

Source: The Report from the "Study Group on the Medical Services in Minamata City and its Surrounding Area"

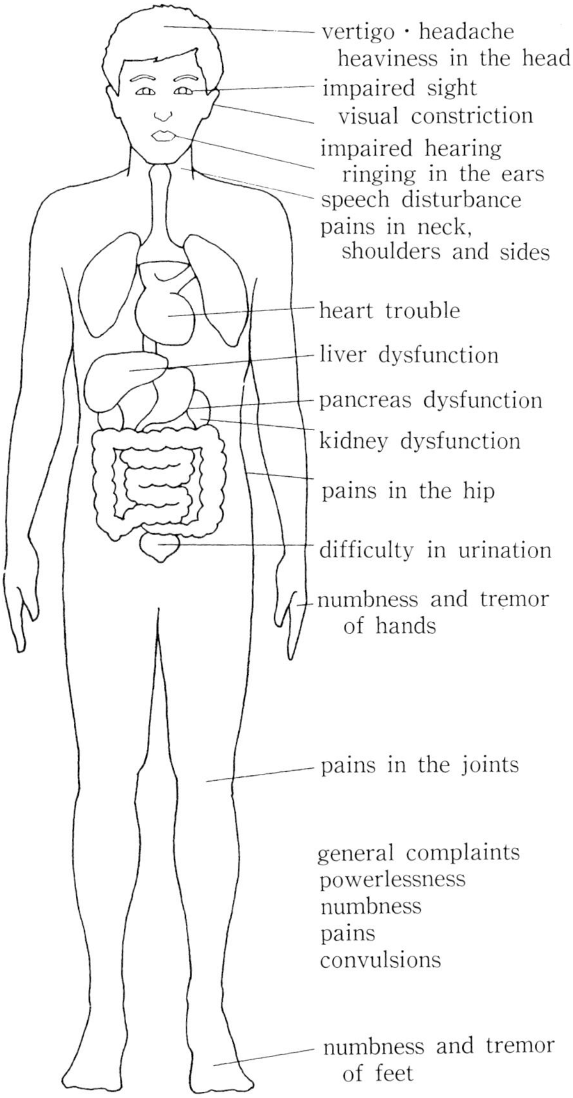

Body diagram labels:
- vertigo · headache, heaviness in the head
- impaired sight, visual constriction
- impaired hearing, ringing in the ears
- speech disturbance
- pains in neck, shoulders and sides
- heart trouble
- liver dysfunction
- pancreas dysfunction
- kidney dysfunction
- pains in the hip
- difficulty in urination
- numbness and tremor of hands
- pains in the joints
- general complaints, powerlessness, numbness, pains, convulsions
- numbness and tremor of feet

Minamata Disease affects the entire body. There is a wide range of symptoms such as the numbness of hands and feet or visual constriction, but there is also a wide variety of invisible health damage such as diabetes induced by liver dysfunction caused by Minamata Disease. Unfortunately a lot of medical practitioners decided these symptoms are not caused by methyl mercury.

DYSGRAPHIA

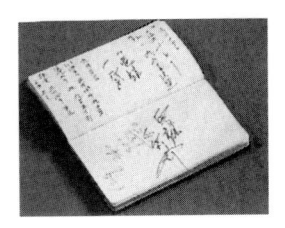

Before he got Minamata Disease

After he got Minamata Disease

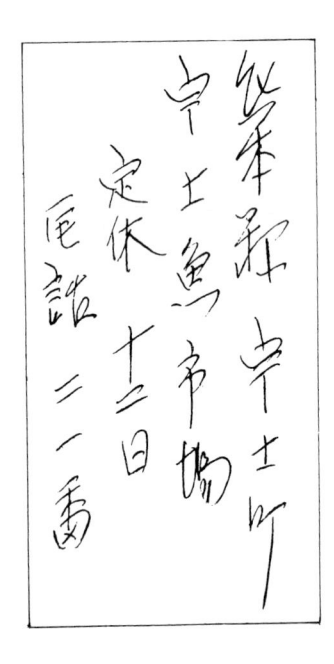

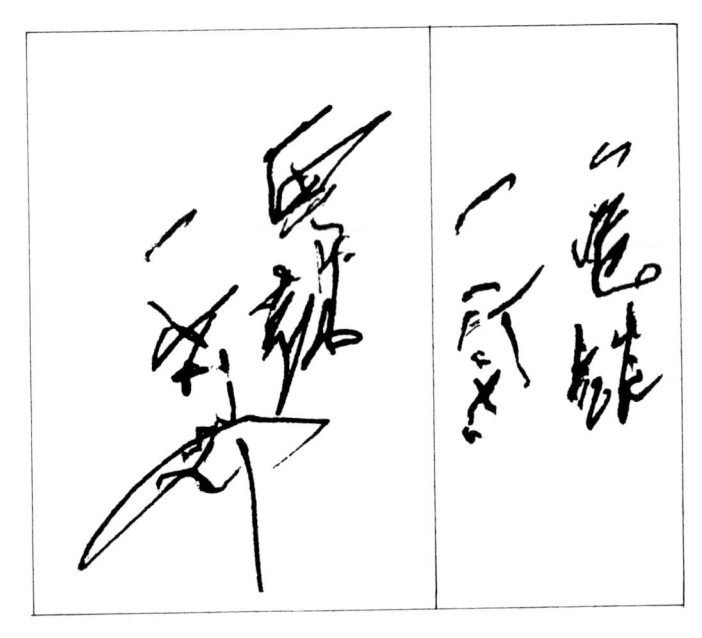

Donated by Fujie Fukuyoshi

    These samples are from a Minamata Disease patient's notebook. His hands tremble when he tries to write. In an advanced stage of the disease, a patient's disability gets worse and what he writes becomes quite beyond recognition compared wtih what he wrote in an earlier stage. This particular patient used to be a fish broker. In 1959 his doctor told him that it was possible that he had got Minamata Disease, so he went into hospital. The members of the fishing co-operative he belonged to, however, compelled him to get out of hospital, insisting that "if we have a Minamata Disease patient in our village, our fish will not sell".

A WIDE RANGE OF DISABILITIES FOR DAILY LIFE

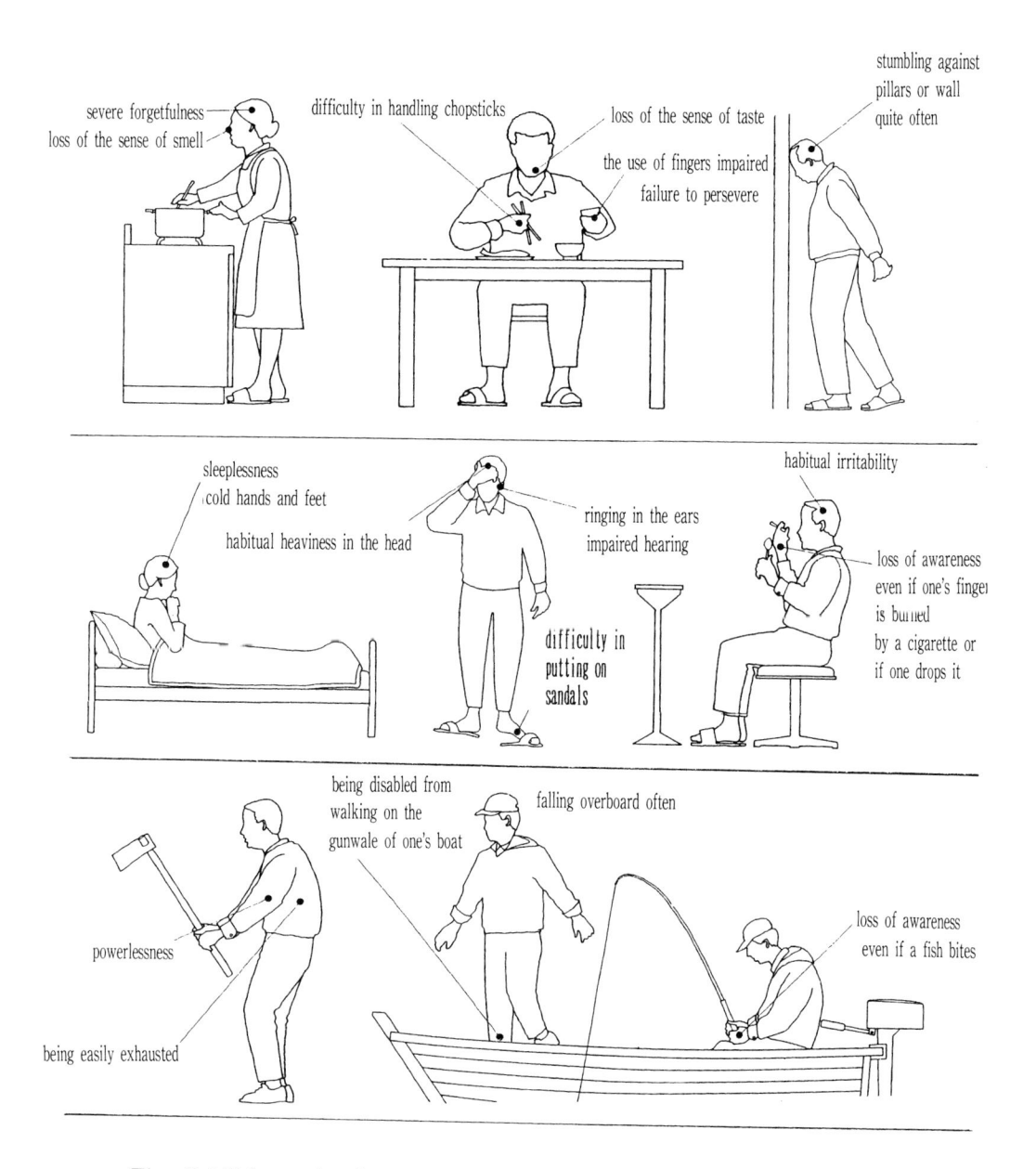

- severe forgetfulness
- loss of the sense of smell
- difficulty in handling chopsticks
- loss of the sense of taste
- the use of fingers impaired
- failure to persevere
- stumbling against pillars or wall quite often
- sleeplessness
- cold hands and feet
- habitual heaviness in the head
- ringing in the ears
- impaired hearing
- difficulty in putting on sandals
- habitual irritability
- loss of awareness even if one's finger is burned by a cigarette or if one drops it
- powerlessness
- being easily exhausted
- being disabled from walking on the gunwale of one's boat
- falling overboard often
- loss of awareness even if a fish bites

The diabilities and pains caused by Minamata Disease have profound implications for the patient's daily life: outwardly invisible disabilities, such as numbness or headaches, pose more than physical problems. For example, if the patient takes rest from his work or takes a day off owing to headaches, he is likely to be branded as a lazy dog. Including such exposure to social injustices, there is no limit to the pains caused by Minamata Disease.

THE ENTIRE SHIRANUI AREA WAS FOUND POLLUTED
——Survey of Mercury Content in the Hair, 1960-1962——

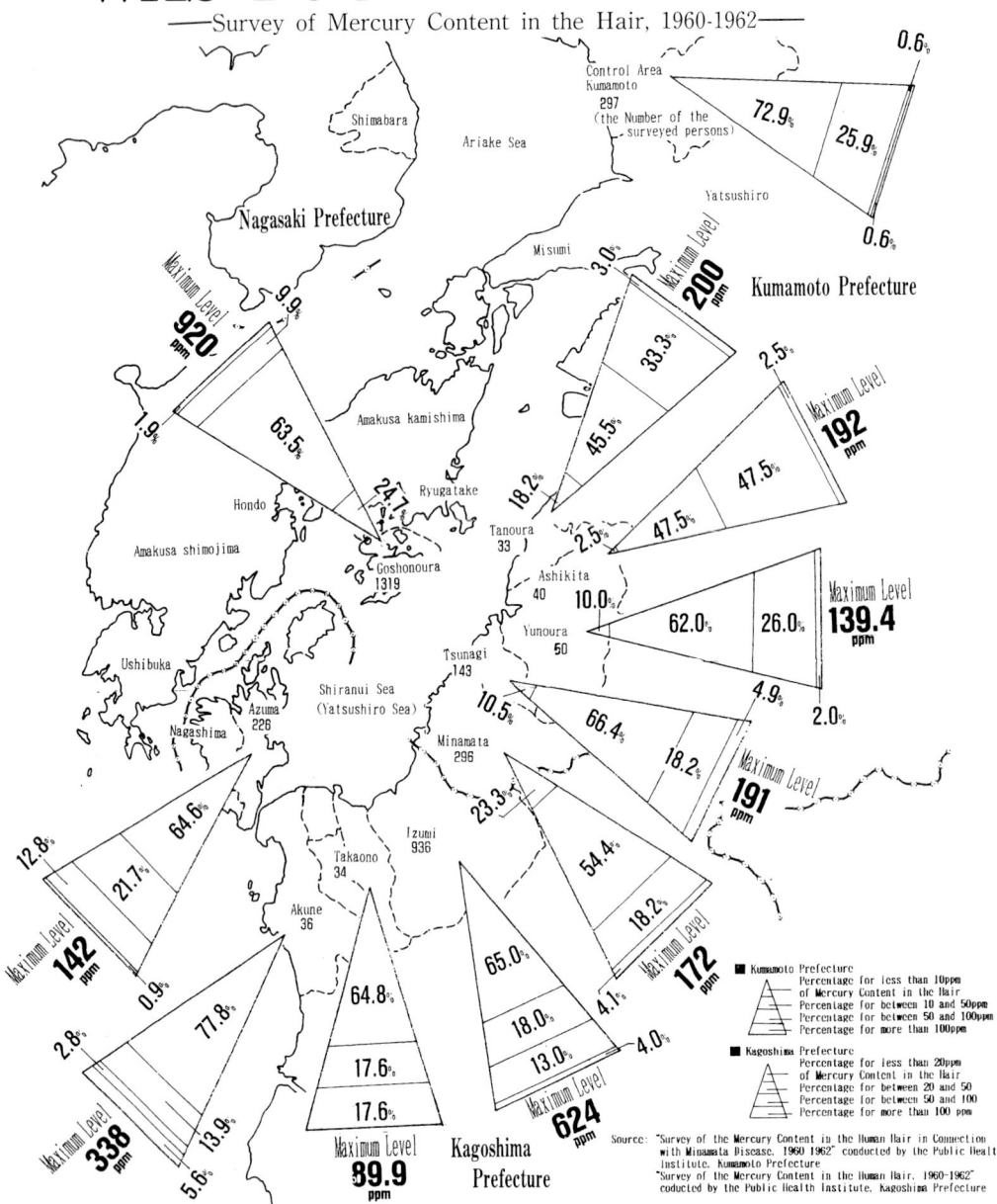

In the early days of Minamata Tragedy (circa. 1960), the local governments of Kumamoto and Kagoshima conducted a survey of the mercury content in the hair of the inhabitants who lived on the Shiranui Sea and found high levels of mercury concentration in the samples. The average level of 1-5ppm is accepted as normal for a healthy Japanese, but somesamples contained up to 920ppm. The outrageous enormity of this figure is quite obvious if compared with that for the control area (Kumamoto City). How unsatisfactory and faulty this survey was may be evident if you see how these findings were not even notified to the inhabitants nvestigated. Chisso was free to pour mercury discharges into the sea.

APPLICATION FOR OFFICIAL CERTIFICATION CAME FROM THE ENTIRE DISTRICT ON THE SHIRANUI SEA

HOW OFFICIAL APPLICANTS HAVE INCREASED

1961

- Ashikita: 2
- Tsunagi: 2
- Minamata (Chisso): 40
- Kagoshima Prefecture: 11

1971

- Yatsushiro: 2
- Tanoura: 2
- Ashikita: 21
- Tsunagi: 46
- Minamata: 231
- Kagoshima Prefecture: 30
- Hondo: 1
- Goshonoura: 2
- Ushibuka: 1

1973

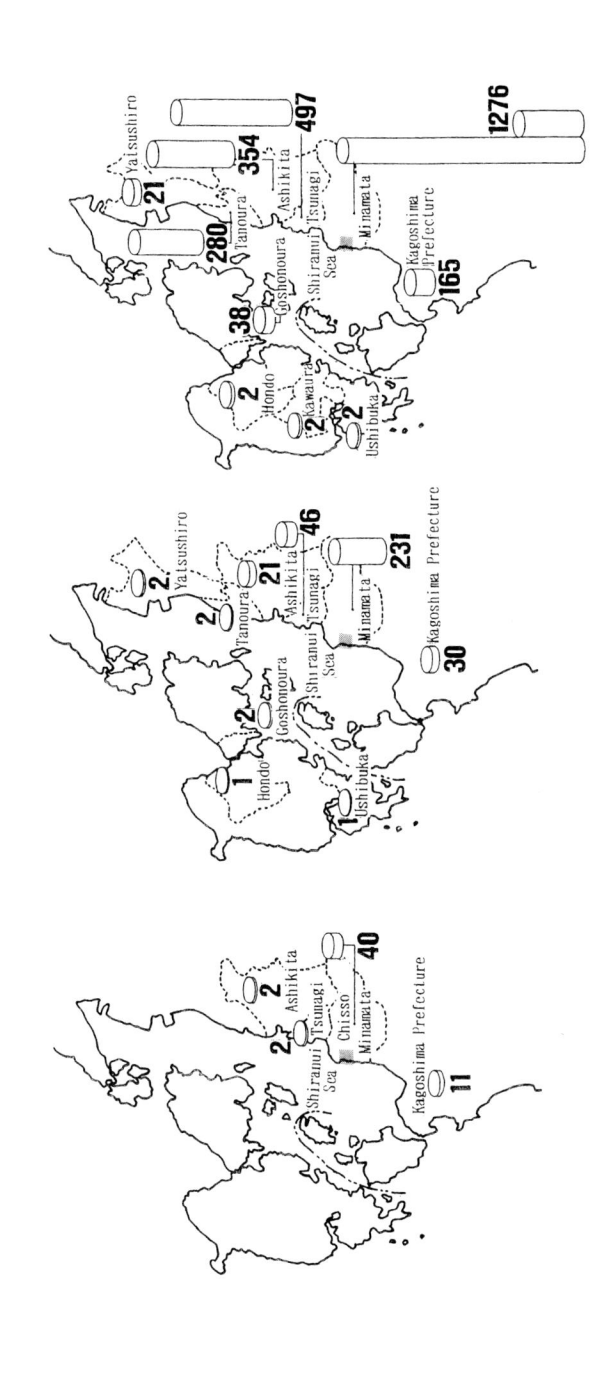

- Yatsushiro: 21
- Tanoura: 280
- Ashikita: 354
- Tsunagi: 497
- Minamata: 1276
- Kagoshima Prefecture: 165
- Goshonoura: 38
- Hondo: 2
- Kawaura: 2
- Ushibuka: 2

Chisso's mercury-contaminated effluents took a heavy toll of those who lived in the entire Shiranui Sea area. What added to the distress of those afflicted by Minamata Disease was the fact that they found themselves helpless, as they were rejected and discriminated against by local inhabitants in their neighbourhood with their prejudice against the disease: they did their best to hide their predicament. Moreover, the local government, hand-in-glove with Chisso and therefore under constraint, would not admit to the presence of the disease. A long series of campaigns organised by patients for recognition and compensation followed, and in due course, Minamata Disease came to be recognised and understood in its true light instead of as a "strange disease". Thus, the patients, "hidden" for long out of public sight, came out into the open to apply for official certification. They came from the entire Shiranui Sea area.

1979

579 · 959 · 65 · 1500 · 790 · 7 · 2 · 5 · 2876 · 1578

1985

1329 · 89 · 2199 · 1164 · 1022 · 13 · 2 · 8 · 3905 · 2928

1990

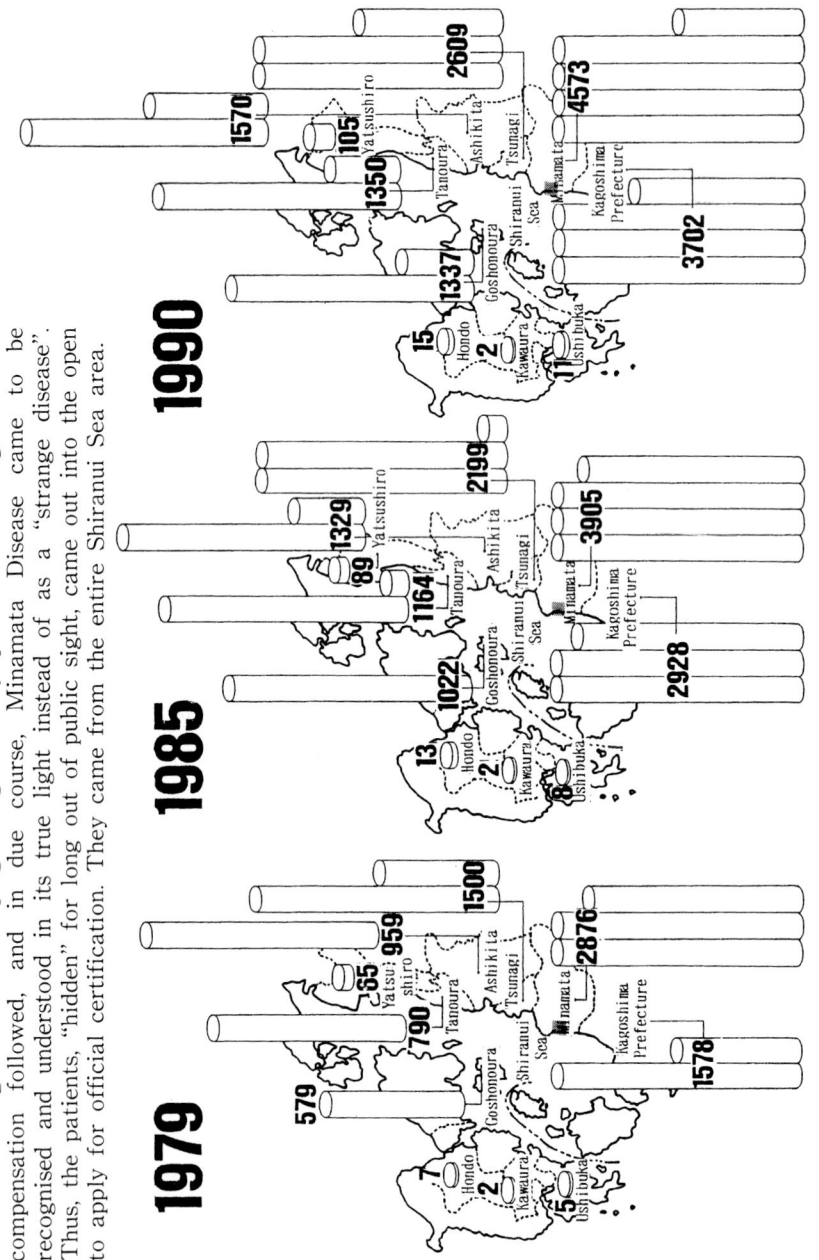

1570 · 105 · 2609 · 1350 · 1337 · 15 · 2 · 11 · 4573 · 3702

MORE THAN 200,000 VICTIMS OF MERCURY POISONING

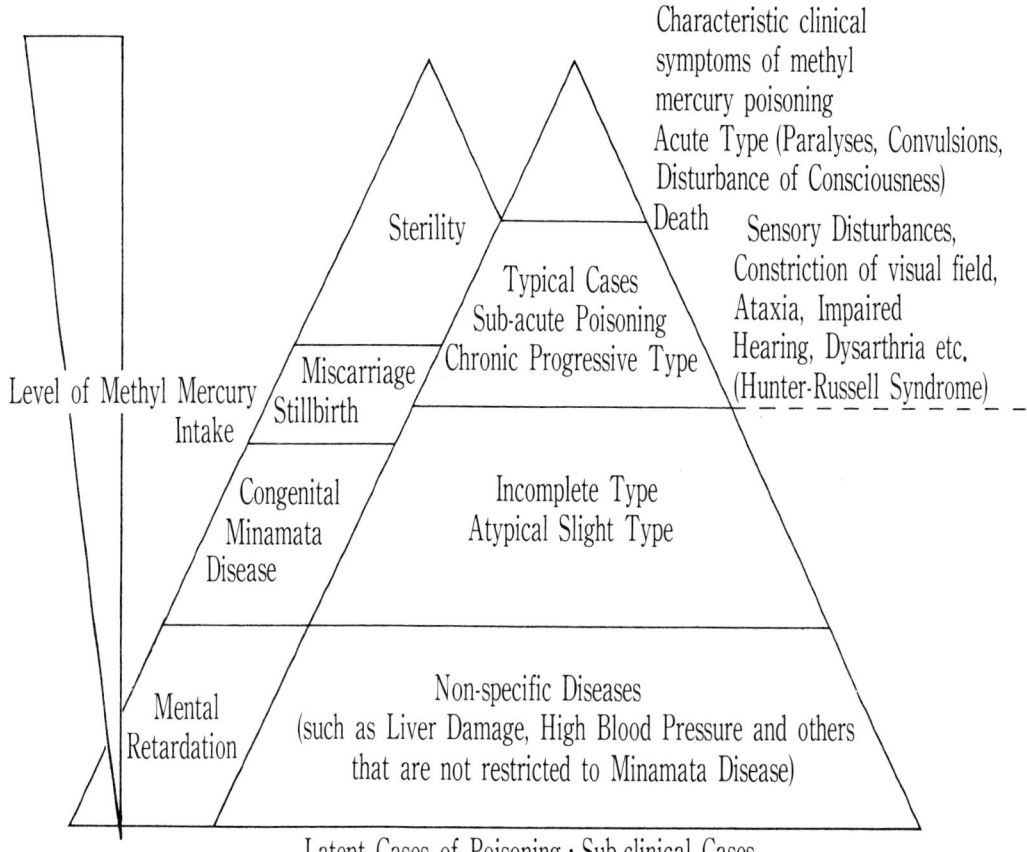

Characteristic clinical symptoms of methyl mercury poisoning

Acute Type (Paralyses, Convulsions, Disturbance of Consciousness)

Death

Sensory Disturbances, Constriction of visual field, Ataxia, Impaired Hearing, Dysarthria etc. (Hunter-Russell Syndrome)

Level of Methyl Mercury Intake

Sterility

Miscarriage Stillbirth

Typical Cases Sub-acute Poisoning Chronic Progressive Type

Congenital Minamata Disease

Incomplete Type Atypical Slight Type

Mental Retardation

Non-specific Diseases (such as Liver Damage, High Blood Pressure and others that are not restricted to Minamata Disease)

Latent Cases of Poisoning · Sub-clinical Cases

In 1940 D.Hunter and D.S.Russell reported cases of methyl mercury poisoning involving workers in an agro-chemical factory in England from which is derived Hunter-Russell Syndrome. The characteristic features are ataxia (disability from writing, walking and so on), sensory disturbances (numbness of hands and feet), impaired hearing (inability to hear), dysarthria (disability from speaking), vision constriction (difficulty in seeing one's surroundings) and tremor. A comparative study of the English cases and those of Minamata led to the discovery in 1959 that Minamata Disease is methyl mercury poisoning. But, unfortunately, it turned out that many Japanese doctors assumed that Minamata Disease was defined by those symptoms alone. As a matter of fact, direct contact with methyl mercury (as was the case in England) produces symptoms which are different from those that occur when the same substance passes through the food chain into man. Minamata Disease, in fact, displays a wide range of different symptoms. There are far more cases of "incomplete", "atypical" or "slight" cases than those that are "typical". Moreover, compared with the healthy inhabitants of other areas, the local residents in Minamata and its surrounding areas reveal a distinct general depletion of physical strength and fitness, which may suggest how large the hidden part of the iceberg may be.

MORE THAN PHYSICAL HEALTH HAS BEEN DAMAGED

Researched by Sadao Togashi and Sadami Maruyama
(Kumamoto University) 1981

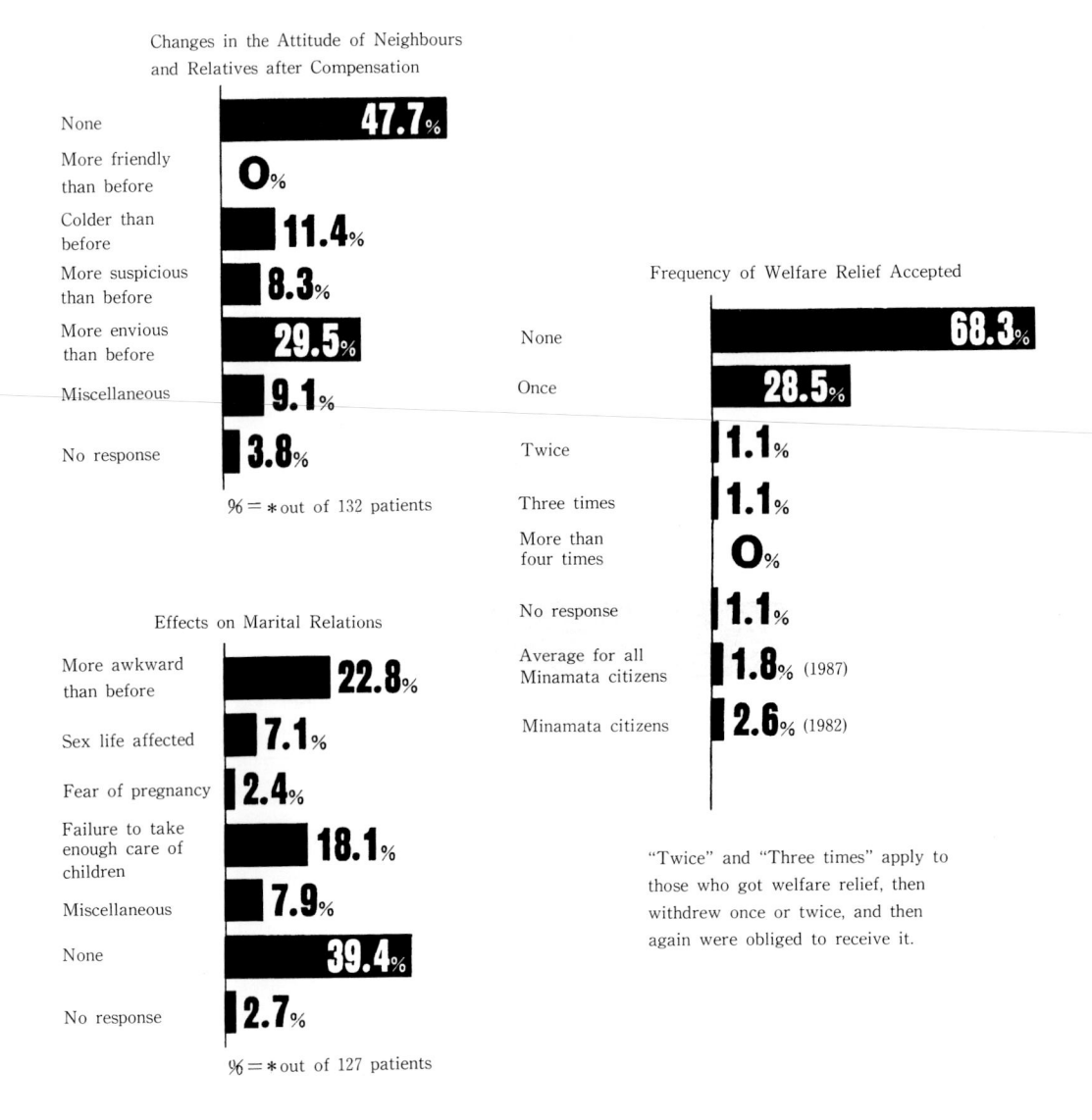

Changes in the Attitude of Neighbours and Relatives after Compensation

- None: 47.7%
- More friendly than before: 0%
- Colder than before: 11.4%
- More suspicious than before: 8.3%
- More envious than before: 29.5%
- Miscellaneous: 9.1%
- No response: 3.8%

% = * out of 132 patients

Effects on Marital Relations

- More awkward than before: 22.8%
- Sex life affected: 7.1%
- Fear of pregnancy: 2.4%
- Failure to take enough care of children: 18.1%
- Miscellaneous: 7.9%
- None: 39.4%
- No response: 2.7%

% = * out of 127 patients

Frequency of Welfare Relief Accepted

- None: 68.3%
- Once: 28.5%
- Twice: 1.1%
- Three times: 1.1%
- More than four times: 0%
- No response: 1.1%
- Average for all Minamata citizens: 1.8% (1987)
- Minamata citizens: 2.6% (1982)

"Twice" and "Three times" apply to those who got welfare relief, then withdrew once or twice, and then again were obliged to receive it.

The victims of Minamata Disease are cursed with grief and anguish at their disability from living and doing as they wish to, in addition to the pains of their physical disabilities. They are disabled from work in the prime of their manhood; they are deliberately shunned by relatives and neighbours; they are excluded from chances of marriage and employment. Chisso still reigns supreme over Minamata City, so its victims still groan and moan under the burden of harm it has inflicted.

THE MEDICAL CARE FOR MINAMATA DISEASE PATIENTS

Source : Sadao Togashi and Sadami Maruyama (Kumamoto University) 1981

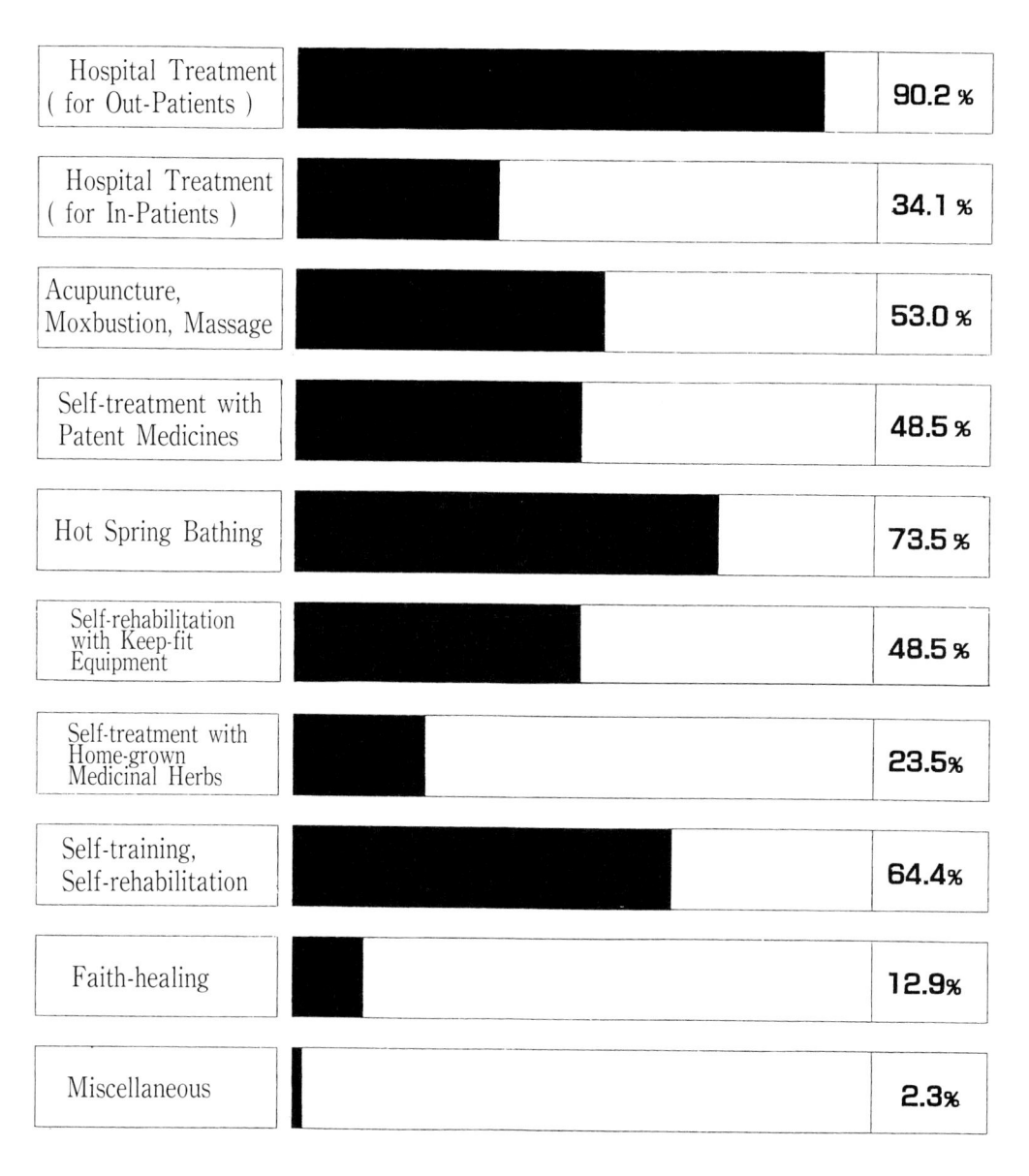

Treatment	Percentage
Hospital Treatment (for Out-Patients)	90.2 %
Hospital Treatment (for In-Patients)	34.1 %
Acupuncture, Moxbustion, Massage	53.0 %
Self-treatment with Patent Medicines	48.5 %
Hot Spring Bathing	73.5 %
Self-rehabilitation with Keep-fit Equipment	48.5 %
Self-treatment with Home-grown Medicinal Herbs	23.5 %
Self-training, Self-rehabilitation	64.4 %
Faith-healing	12.9 %
Miscellaneous	2.3 %

Most patients are now suffering from the added pains and anguish of progressing symptoms and old age. It is widely believed that "Minamata Disease is incurable", and dozens of years have passed since the onset of the disease. But they have been trying their best to alleviate as much of their daily sufferings as they could. They are still trying every possible means of recovery such as going to hospital or buying remedial equipment.

THE SCOPE AND DEPTH OF DAMAGE AND SUFFERINGS

The victims of Minamata Disease have suffered more than physical damage. They are not only ill but they have also lost the sea contaminated and killed by Chisso's toxic effluents. The sea used to give Minamata fishermen something to live for as well as their livelihood. Moreover, the "strange disease" or the "contagious disease" (as Minamata Disease was once called) set them apart: they were ostracised and discriminated against, which was quite unjustifiable. This did not only apply to adult patiets but also to children who were denied schooling or to young people who found themselves deprived of chances of employment or marriage. Such an aggravating combination of health damage, economic and social deprivation and discrimination has often led to the breakdown of the family and home. Thus, Minamata Disease has destroyed the whole of the victim's life.

MINAMATA DISEASE VICTIMS CONDEMNED BY POLITICIANS

"The Certification Committee is having much trouble in telling the real thing from the false. Some people are judged as having no problem with their vision when applying for a driving licence but at a medical check-up they say their vision is constricted".

Kunio Sugimura, Member of Kumamoto Prefectural Assembly (Chairman of the Special Committee for the Prevention of Environmental Pollution, M.D.) 1975

"Many of the applicants for certification are false patients bent on compensation. They are all for grubbing money".

Ichiro Saisho, Member of Kumamaoto Prefectural Assembly (representative of Minamata City), 1975

"In Kumamoto people apply for certification and get money. I suppose all the inhabitants of Kumamoto will soon be certified as patients of Minamata Disease. I too wish to live in Kumamoto and be certified as one".

Yasushi Morishita, Member of the Upper House (Chairman of the Environment Sub-committee, Liberal-Democratic Party), 1979

"I understand that the people we met just now at Meisui-en have rather low I.Q.. But these letters are written very well or in a certain style. I wonder if those girls have really written them".

Shintaro Ishiwara, Director General of the Environment Agency, 1977

Both the certified patients and those applying for certification have been steadily exposed to a long catalogue of bad language and condemnation by politicians, both at local and national levels, who ought to be on the side of the victims. Public comments of the kind listed above, coming from men of political bias and influence, have had adverse effects on public opinion and added to the burden of prejudice and discrimination under which Minamata victims have been labouring.

THE KIND OF MUD FLUNG AT MINAMATA VICTIMS BY LOCAL PEOPLE

Those who have got compensation have made a lot of money by lying in bed.

That one is a patient of the strange disease.

Disgusting!

The newspapers are making mountains out of mole-hills.

You don't want to work here any more. A lazy dog like you.

He is always saying he is a patient, but he won the gold medal at the athletic meet.

What a gang of conceited beggars!

He used to lie in bed, but, now certified, he is riding a motor-bike.

They are practising how to totter about in order to get certified.

In fact, they are alcoholics.

A pack of paupers are begging the Company for alms.

What a shame! How you want money so!

Compensation has made a new gang of millionaires, and they have made the land prices rise from 3,000 yen per 3.3m² to 50,000.

Don't batten on our taxes!

They deserve the strange disease, for they have eaten weakened fish.

Some people have deliberately chosen to eat rotten fish.

Keep off our premises! You stand in the way of other customers.

What are you here at school for?

Keep off! It's contagious!

Thanks to the patients, nobody will buy our fish.

The light has gone out of our town because of the patients.

What are you doing? A pack of fools!

Many of them are certified, but all of them are working all right.

In the early days of Minamata Disease, the patients' complaints were given such misleading names as the "strange disease" or the "contagious disease"; even brothers or sisters and relatives gave them a wide berth.

A long struggle led to Chisso's agreement to pay damages to the patients in 1973, but, unfortunately, compensation has created a new wave of malicious slander and envy, to add to the patients' grief and anguish. In the early 1970s, when many new patients came forward and applied for official certifi-cation, they had the name of "fake patients" hurled at them. Thus, they were the centre of cruel and grim attention, further fed by "ignorance" (based on the assumption that deformed hands and feet are the only signs of Minamata Disease) and by "prejudice" (i.e. "They want compensation, so they will tell lies").

All the people who have eaten the fish from the Shiranui Sea are poisoned——that is a hard fact, and that is the "crime" that Chisso has committed. It is not until these two facts are understood in their true light that unjustifiable harsh language will cease to be used against the patients of Minamata Disease.

3

A LONG STRUGGLE

THIRTY YEARS OF VICTIMISATION AND SUFFERING

SEARCH FOR THE CAUSE AND SOURCE OF MINAMATA DISEASE

At first Minamata Disease was labelled as a "strange disease". Its presence was first reported in 1956 by Dr.Hosokawa, and, in 1959, a research team of the Kumamoto University Medical School found that it is caused by an intake of fish contaminated by Chisso's toxic effluents. Deprived of the source of their livelihood, the fishermen found themselves reduced to the extremes of poverty and distress so that a couple of thousands of them got together and invaded the premises of Chisso factory complex, demanding an immediate cessation of toxic wastes discharged. They were only rewarded with small sums of money which were supposed to compensate them for damage to fishing. Not only the discovery of mercury as the cause of the disease but also the identification of Chisso's effluents as the source of mercury poisoning failed to persuade Chisso to acknowledge responsibility for Minamata Disease and to pay damages to its victims. Compensation and relief were replaced by *Mimaikin* (payments in token of one's sympathy or pity): e.g. an annual payment of ten thousand yen to an adult victim who is alive.

The cause and source of Minamata Disease was left unacknowledged. It was also officially assumed that there were no more patients. Mercury was being discharged into the sea while nothing was done about it.

THE CATS WERE THE FIRST TO GO MAD AND DIE
—1954—

ALL CATS KILLED BY EPILEPSY
Local residents of Modo overwhelmed by mice and rats

On July 31, T.Ishimoto, Modo Hamlet, reported to the Public Health Section of Minamata City and complained that recently there had appeared a large army of mice and rats in Modo and that there were so many of them around that the local residents did not know what to do.

Modo is a small hamlet of 120 fishermen. Something strange happened in early June: their cats went mad and died of what they called epilepsy. Nearly all of them (the original number being more than one hundred) have died, and the local residents are plagued by swarms of rats and mice that will play (there being no cats) and do what they like with people's property. Some of them were in a hurry to bring new cats in, but these, too, went spinning round and round and died. Being at the end of their tether, they decided to appeal to the city authorities.

They have no rice fields in Modo area, so pesticides are assumed to be irrelevant. Nobody knows what to make of this strange and weird phenomenon, but the Public Health Section is now ready to tackle the rats and mice.

It had started a year before: fish, birds and cats were seen to die an unnatural death. All the cats disappeared in Modo. This is the first report of something being wrong with the ecology of the Shiranui Sea.

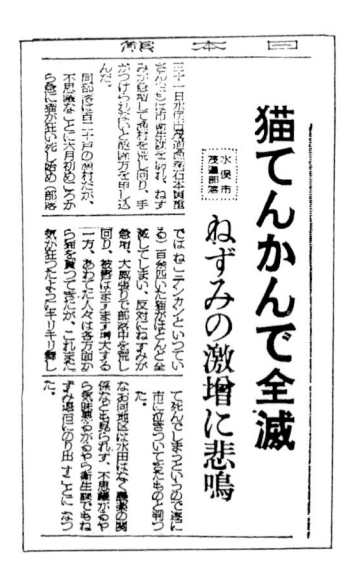

MINAMATA DISEASE WAS DISCOVERED
—1956—

Official Report from Director of Public Health Office, Minamata

Title: On the Strange Infant Disease that Occurred in Tsukiura, Minamata

Date: 4 May 1956

to the Head of the Public Health Division, Kumamoto Prefecture

On 1 May the paediatrician of the Chisso Factory Hospital, Minamata, reported a strange infant disease that occurred in Tsukiura area. The results of our investigaion are as follows.

1. Patient: T.S., aged 6
   She had a slight fever and other cold-like symptoms at the end of March this year. Around 14 April, she developed a stiffness and numbness of limbs, was sleepless and crying all night, had no appetiteexcept for a bottle of Yakult a day, and became gradually enfeebled. She was hospitalised at the Department of Paediatrics of Chisso Hospital. It was found that she was stiff and numb in the limbs and disturbed in speech. Being unable to ingest food since hospitalisation, she has had an infusion of nutriments through the nostrils; her temperature has remained normal nearly all the time; and she has been torpid and apathetic.
   Laboratory check-up: exacerbated patellar reflex; Babinski's reflex (+); Körnig reflex (—); no stiffness in the neck; the spinal fluids are watery and transparent; Pandy's test (—); number of cells in the spinal fluids is 3.
   This patient is the most seriously afflicted.
2. Patient: T.J., aged 3
   She shares most of the symptoms that S., her sister, has, but they are not so serious as to need hospitalisation.
3. Patient: M.F., aged 7, who lives in the first patient's neighbourhood.
   How it started, as told by her mother on 2 May.
   On 11 April, she was diagnosed as afflicted with polio by Dr.Ichikawa, Fukuro, Minamata.
   On 16 April, she was diagnosed as a case of malnutrition at the paediatric department, Minamata Municipal Hospital.
   On 17 April, she was diagnosed as a case of cerebral palsy by Dr. Ukichi, Minamata.
   Since then she has been undergoing examination as an out-patient at the paediatric department of Chisso Factory Hospital. Her principal symptom is a stiffness and numbness of limbs which is gradually progressing.

Additional Remarks:
As for T.S. her eyesight is also beginning to fail to such an extent that she finds it difficult to see hand movements at a distance of 20cm but they are easily recognisable at 50cm. Dr.Tanigawa (ophthalmologist) fears that she may develop an atrophy of the optic nerves.

Direct information from S's mother on similar cases in their neighbourhood.

1. Their cat, and other cats in their neighbourhood, were thrown into convulsions and died one after another. It started in January this year. About ten days after the onset of the disease, all of them jumped into the fire, the water or the sea and died. There were five or six of them in all.
2. Of the three children of Mr.Yonemori, a six-year-old boy was diagnosed as a case of polio last July. His hands are twisted and stiffened now.
3. A seven-year-old girl of E., their next-door neighbour, is afflicted with symptoms similar to those of S. It started a few days ago.
4. K.S., another neighbour aged about 55, lost the movement of his feet two years ago and,then,that of his hands. He became unable to speak and finally went mad. He is now in a mental hospital in Kumamoto.
5. Y.K., another neighbour in the third grade of elementary school, was diagnosed as a case of polio at Oda Clinic, Minamata and died. His uncle, who took care of him, was soon afflicted with similar symptoms and died.

The occurrence of the disease in the families in the same neighbourhood who share the same well may indicate the presence of some toxic substance in the water of the well. We took some samples of the water and sent them to the Prefectural Public Health Research Centre.

An official report was made to the Public Health Office, Minamata, by Dr.Hosokawa and others on some of the patients who visited Chisso Hospital: they were described as "cases without any precedent". That was the day when Minamata Disease was officially discovered: 1 May 1956. Immediately an extensive epidemiological survey was conducted by a team of health officers from the Public Health Office, doctors from Minamata Municipal Hospital and local medical practitioners on the inhabitants of the hamlets along the coast of Minamata Bay. A surprisingly large number of patients were discovered, even in small hamlets, so that all of them were suspected of some unknown contagious disease and put into an isolation ward. Later, the theory of infection and contagion was dismissed as the research group of the Medical School, Kumamoto University, decided that Minamata Disease is caused by the mercury in Chisso's waste discharges. It is quite unfortunate, however, that the initial stigma of a "contagious" or "dirty" disease still clings to the patients who are groaning under the weight of layer upon layer of unjustifiable prejudice and discrimination.

NOTHING WAS DONE ABOUT THE CONTAMINATED FISH —1957—

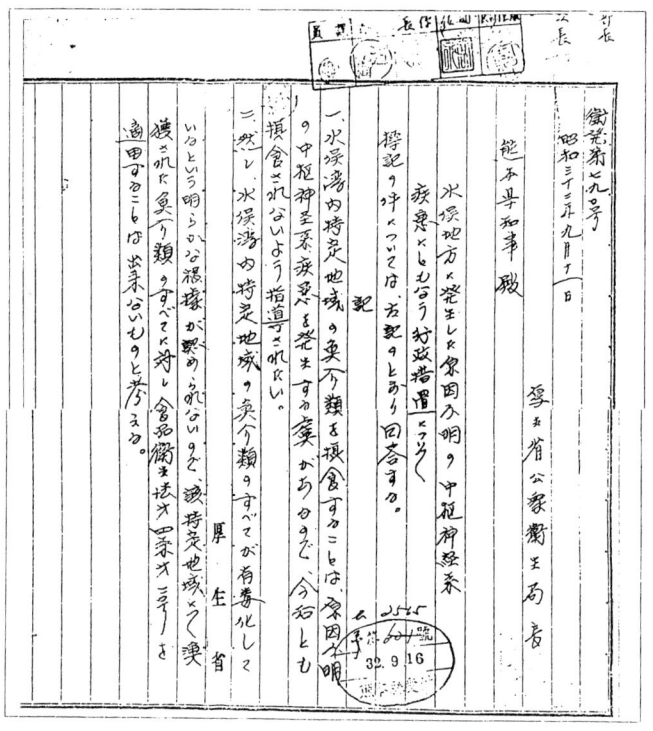

The Official Notification (No.790)　Date: 11 September 1957　From: Director of the Public Health Bureau, Welfare Ministry　To: Governor of Kumamoto Prefecture

Title: On the administrative measures to be taken in connection with the unknown disease of the central nervous system that has occurred in Minamata

Our official reply to the above question is as follows:
1. We recommend that you should continue your policy of warning against the ingestion of fish and shellfish caught in a specified area of Minamata Bay because it may lead to the occurrence of the unknown disease of the central nervous system.
2. But there is no clear evidence that all the fish and shellfish in the specified area are poisoned. Therefore, we have decided that it is impossible to apply Provision 4-2 of the Food Sanitation Act to all the fish and shellfish to be caught in that area.

　It was gradually becoming clear that people got ill when they ate the fish and shellfish caught in Minamata Bay, but the Ministry of Welfare did not decide against catching them.
　Never since then has there been any legislative or administrative action taken against catching fish and shellfish in Minamata Bay——though the fishermen themselves imposed a voluntary ban on fishing in the Bay in 1960. But the fishery co-operative lifted the embargo in 1964, believing that "nothing is wrong". The fish and shellfish continued to be caught and eaten by local people until the outbreak of the third Minamata Disease in 1973 when a voluntary restriction was again imposed.

FISHERMEN ROSE IN PROTEST
—1959—

RESOLUTION : Yunoura Fishery Co-operative 30 September 1959

1. Chisso should discontinue its release of effluents until facilities for treatment and purification are completed.
2. Chisso should remove the slimy sludge at Hyakken port and along the Hachiman coast.
3. A scientific investigation should be conducted into the pollution of the Shiranui Sea due to Chisso's industrial discharges.
4. Relief measures should be taken to help fishermen, such as financing a switchover to other types of fishing.

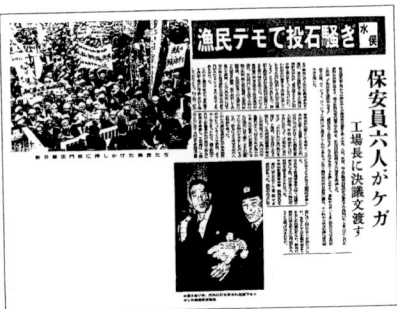

Fishermen Demonstrate and Throw Stones : Minamata
    Six security men injured
    Resolution handed to Factory Director
        ——Kumamoto Daily News 18 October 1959

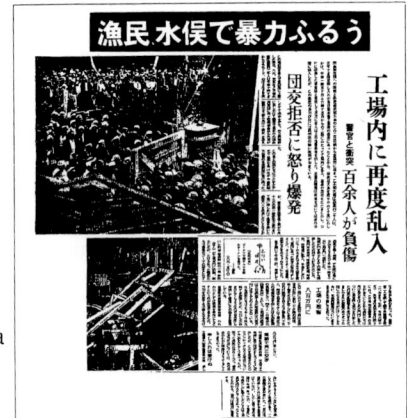

1,500 Fishermen Crashed the Gate : Chisso, Minamata
    Seven security men injured
    Fishermen demand cessation of operations
——Kumamoto Daily News 3 November 1959

Damage to fishing operations in the Shiranui Sea goes back to the early days of Chisso's foundation in Minamata. In 1925, for example, Minamata fishermen demanded compensation from Chisso.

All the fishermen who lived on the Shiranui Sea suffered from Chisso's waste effluents : there were few fish to catch and there were few people to buy their fish if they caught some. In 1959 they organised a large demonstration and swarmed into the Chisso premises, demanding damages but they were rewarded with some of them being arrested by the police.

Chisso would not acknowledge their industrial wastes being the cause of Minamata Disease, as was confirmed by the experimental cat No.400. They managed to get away with it, condescending to mete out a nominal compensation of 100 million yen and tactful enough to provide against "the patients' right to additional compensation even if their effluents were to be verified later as the cause of Minamata Disease". It was the cessation of their industrial wastes that the Minamata fishermen, and patients as well, demanded.

THE PATIENTS ROUSED TO ACTION AT LAST
—1959—

RESOLUTION

To Mr.Eiichi Nishida
    Director
    Minamata Factory, Chisso

It is generally accepted that Minamata Disease, which broke out in about 1953, is caused by your waste effluents and has taken a heavy toll of the life and health of local residents. Therefore, we, 78 victims, demand 234,000,000 yen for compensation. We also demand that your reply should come by 30 November.

25 November 1959
Eizo Watanabe
President

Friendly Association of Minamata Disease Patients and their Families

---

ASSOCIATION MEMBERS SIT-IN
The Factory says "No"
Nishi-Nippon Shimbun 1 December 1959

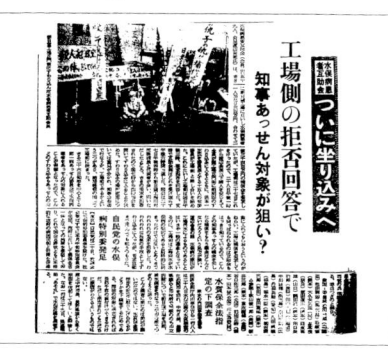

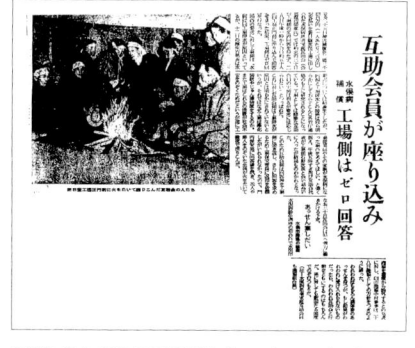

SIT-IN PROTEST by Association members
In protest against the Director's "No"
With a view to the Governor's intecerssion?
Kumamoto Daily News 29 November 1959

    In the early days of Minamata Disease, which was called the "strange disease" or "yoi-yoi" (a popular name for locomotor ataxia), its victims avoided public attention and lived in humble obscurity, until in 1957 they organised themselves into an association of Minamata Disease patients and their families for mutual assistance, and, two years later, they plucked up their heart to take action against Chisso and demanded compensation. They found themselves helpless and got no support in Chisso-dominated Minamata. If you were to rise against the lord and master of your town, you should be prepared to get ostracised by the whole town.

CHISSO'S FRAUDULENT CONTRACT
—1959—

(MIMAIKIN) CONTRACT

Article 4 A (i.e. Chisso) is to stop its payments of Mimaikin if and when (i.e. in the very month when the following decision is taken) it is decided that Minamata Disease is not caused by A's waste discharges.

Article 5 B (i.e. the patients) relinquish their calim to further compensation even if it is decided that Minamata Disease is caused by A's waste discharges.

    Evidently this was a case of fraud. Chisso knew (but would not acknowledge) the fact that Minamata Disease is caused by their toxic wastes and deliberately substituted "Mimaikin for poor people" (payments in token of one's sympathy or pity for poor people) for proper compensation for murder and injury. Deceased victims were awarded 300,000 yen, with an annual pension of 100,000 yen for adults and 10,000 for children who were alive. This agreement on Mimaikin was later to be annulled by a court ruling (1973) as violating public order and morals. Such is the enormity of Chisso's imposition on the patients' innocence that they were forced to accept that "they relinquish their claim to further compensation even if the factory is found responsible for the disease".

THE PATIENTS' CAMPAIGN SWUNG INTO HIGH GEAR

The outbreak of Niigata Minamata Disease in 1965 finally brought the national government round to the official recognition in 1968 that "Chisso is to blame for Minamata Disease". Unfortunately, however, the Friendly Association of Minamata Disease Patients and their Families was split later because of differences of opinion as to what policy to take in their struggle for proper compensation. The Law-suit faction decided to take legal action in 1969. Those were the days of public opinion all against environmental pollution, which favoured the patients' active movement that followed. Another group of "new patients", who were certified in October 1971, launched a long series of "independent negotiations" with Chisso. The favourable court ruling in March 1973 and the patients' follow-up negotiations, accompanied by sit-ins and demonstrations, finally led to the signing of the Compensation Agreement in June 1973 which provides for all the officially certified patients.

THE COURT RULING ON MINAMATA DISEASE

—Part of the Reasons for the Decision—

"Chemical firms, when discharging their waste effluents out of their premises, should primarily provide for maximum safety by employing expertise and technology of the highest level available in investigating their quality for possible toxic substances as well as for possible adverse effects on the life and health of animals, plants and man. If their wastes are found to be toxic, or if there is any doubt as to their safety, the firms should adopt the most effective preventive measures required, including the immediate cessation of operations. Especially, in cases where the life and health of local residents is involved, it is their highest responsibility and obligation to prevent any possible health damage."

"This is simply because no firm should be allowed to injure and sacrifice the life and health of local residents."

"Granting that the quality of the defendant's waste effluents happened to meet the statutory requirements for safety or those recommended by the government and that they were better treated at his premises than elsewhere, there is sufficient evidence for the inference that the defendant was consistently at fault in discharging toxic effluents from the acetaldehyde plant. The release of wastes was inseparable from the defendant's production activities as a whole. Therefore, the defendant should be held responsible for professional negligence."

"The defendant's basic policy of 'Profit first and human life last' is most responsible for the outbreak of Minamata Disease."

KUMAMOTO DISTRICT COURT
20 March 1973

COMPENSATION AGREEMENT
—1973—

AGREEMENT

In order to solve the problems of Minamata Disease, such as compensation for the patients and their families, the Tokyo Negotiation Group of Minamata Disease Patients and the Chisso Corporation have agreed to the following stipulations.

Preamble

1. Chisso Corporation unreservedly admits that their Minamata factory has contaminated Minamata Bay and its neighbouring areas extending as far as to Amakusa by discharging waste effluents containing toxic substances and that consequently they have caused a disastrous Minamata Disease which destroys man and his life.
2. Chisso Corporation is sincerely ashamed of their failure to make adequate efforts, even after the official discovery of Minamata Disease in 1956, to prevent fatal damage from spreading, to investigate its possible causes, or to relieve the patients' sufferings, with the result of increased contamination and suffering. Chisso is also ashamed of their stubbornly uncooperative attitude in solving the problems of Minamata Disease even after the causative substance and source were dentified and those problems were brought to public attention.
3. Chisso Corporation sincerely apologises to the patients and their families for their sufferings and deprivations due to Minamata Disease, for the mental pains inflicted by Chisso's irresponsible attitude and for the accumulation of humiliations and discriminations piled upon their heads by the local community.
Chisso Corporation also sincerely apologises to society as a whole for their deliberate evasion of responsibility and for their reluctance to settle the problems of Minamata Disease, because Chisso is responsible for the confusion and panic into which the whole nation has now been thrown by the outbreak of a third Minamata Disease.
4. Kumamoto District Court has found that Minamata Disease is caused by Chisso's industrial effluents, thereby confirming their gross negligence and granting the plaintiffs' claim to compensation. Chisso Corporation agrees to accept this ruling and fulfill all of its provisions.
5. After the signing of the "Mimaikin" contract, Chisso Corporation decided that Minamata Disease was over: hence their failure to acknowledge the presence of patients not only in Minamata and its neighbourhood but in the whole Shiranui Sea area or to look for latent patients.
That is why the whole extent and depth of Minamata Disease is yet to be explored even now. Chisso Corporation acknowledges their responsibility for these latent patients and agrees to endeavour to find and relieve them.
6. Chisso Corporation agrees to confirm their determination to make no more mistakes and to prevent any more contamination and pollution.They also agree to provide relevant information on request in a consistent effort to dissipate any anxiety and misgivings on the part of local residents. As to the clean-up operations of the contaminated waters of Minamata Bay and its neighbourhood, Chisso Corporation agrees to make a joint action plan with the ministries concerned and the local governments and to implement it as soon as possible. Chisso Corporation also agrees to conclude an agreement for the prevention of pollution with the local authorities concerned as soon as possible.
7. Chisso Corporation agrees to take immediate and concrete measures for the relief and welfare of patients and their families, planned and adjusted in such a way to meet their specific requirements, such as those for medical care, physical rehabilitation, social rehabilitation and re-employment.
8. Chisso Corporation extends their regret and apology to the Tokyo Negotiation Group of Minamata Disease Patients for their uncooperative attitude during the negotiations and for the delayed settlement for which Chisso alone is responsible.

COMPENSATION AWARDS AS THEY STAND NOW
—9 January 1991—

Chisso Pays

		A	B	C
Solatia to Patients		18,000,000yen	17,000,000yen	16,000,000yen
Solatia to Patients' Relatives	Spouse	4,5~6,000,000	3,500,000	
	Parents and Children	1,0~3,000,000	1,000,000	
Special Life-long Adjustment Allowance		146,000	76,000	56,000

○ Medical Expenses: the total payment for illnesses connected with Minamata Disease (all complications and accidents due to Minamata Disease)
○ Medical Allowances:

to Hospitalised Patients	for more than 15 days	for 8-14 days	within 7 days
	31,000yen	29,100yen	21,800yen
to Out-patients	for more than 8 days	for 2-7 days	
	21,800	19,800	

○ Nursing Care Allowance   40,500yen per month
○ Funeral Expenses   474,000yen
○ Hot Spring Treatment: 4 overnight trips and 32 day trips a year
○ Expenses for Acupuncture and Moxibustion: the Total Sum

※ Sliding Scale: Special adjustment allowances and Funeral expenses are revised once in two years (but once a year in cases where the index of the previous year exceeds that of the year before last by more than 5%)
※ Medical Expenses, Medical Care and Nursing Care Allowances conform to those provided by Pollution Relief Fund Act.

FUND PAYS

the Fund for the Livelihood and Medical Relief of Minamata Disease Patients provided by Chisso and entrusted with the Kumamoto branch of the Japan Red Cross. The following allowances come from the interests on the Fund.
○ Allowance for Diapers: 10,000 yen per month
○ Nursing Allowance: 19,000 yen per month
○ Incense Money: 100,000 yen
○ Schooling Assistance for Congenital Cases: 50,300 yen annually for elementary school children and 74,100 yen annually for junior high school children
○ Massage Expenses: 1,000 yen for one treatment; up to 25 treatments in a year
○ Expenses for travelling to hospital: one trip a day

Up to 10km	10-20km	More than 20km	Isolated islands
270 yen	400 yen	600 yen	680 yen

A long spell of law-suits and independent negotiations finally succeeded in forcing Chisso to make some compensation. The agreement was signed on 9 July 1973, according to which Chisso has been paying damages to officially certified patients.

DIRECT NEGOTIATIONS WITH CHISSO PRESIDENT

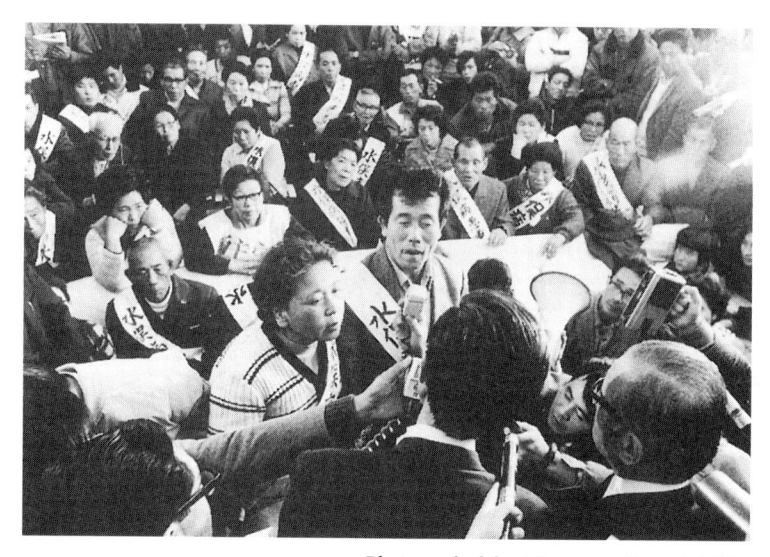

Photographed by Miyamoto Narumi 1973

Patients of the Law-suit faction and those of the Independent Negotiation faction were united into the Tokyo Negotiation Group. They started direct negotiations.

PATIENTS OF THE INDEPENDENT NEGOTIATION FACTION SIT-IN

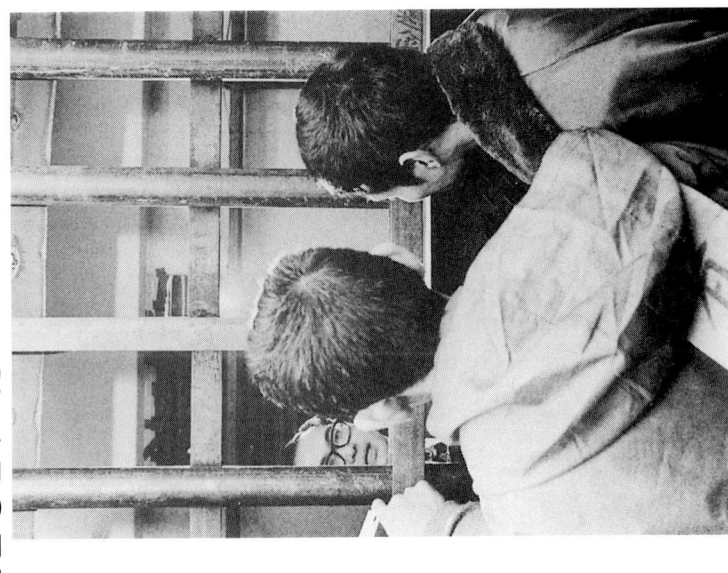

Photographed by Miyamoto Narumi 19

Photographed by Miyamoto Narumi 1973

A few patients, whose applications for official certification were rejected by Kumamoto prefectural authorities, filed a formal complaint to the Environment Agency against this administrative act. The Agency, founded in '71, accepted their complaint and decided that "Kumamoto prefecture should be free to certify those whose eligibility could not be denied". Chisso, however, refused to deal with those patients newly certified by the "1971 decision by the Environment Agency", insisting that they were of a different category from the old certified ones. Those "new" patients, including their leader, Teruo Kawamoto, resorted to sit-in tactics, demanding direct negotiations with Chisso for compensation. They asserted that "one man's life is as precious as another's" and asked Chisso for 30,000,000 hen for each patient. Most of the Minamata citizens turned their back on their just demand.

ORGANISED SUPPORT OF THE VICTIMS

There had been no organised support for Minamata Disease patients for a long time until a little before they filed a compensation suit against Chisso in June 1969. The first voluntary organisation in support of the victims was the Citizens' Council for Countering Minamata Disease formed by Minamata volunteers in January 1968. Minamata was generally dominated by Chisso, so that it took just as much bracing-up and determination to support the victims as it took the latter to rise against Chisso. This first group, however, paved the way for a second supportive "Organisation for the Indictment of Minamata Disease" set up in Kumamoto City in April 1969 and for more similar groups to be formed in Tokyo, Osaka and elsewhere in the years that followed, joined by non-political citizens recruited from the emerging students' movements of the day and intellectuals. These supporters were then in attendance and assistance, at court ,at the table of direct negotiations or on victims' farms or in their fishing-boats. They also assisted in raising funds for the patients' campaigns. Quite a few of them were encouraged to join by Michiko Ishimure's *Paradise in the Sea of Sorrow* (1969) and Noriaki Tsuchimoto's film *Minamata Disease——The Victims and Their World* (1971). The Second and the Third Court Trials, defended by a group of sympathetic lawyers, are supported by progressive political parties and trade unions.

PATIENTS' STRUGGLE AGAINST THE CERTIFICATION SYSTEM

A series of court trials on Minamata Disease and the outbreak of a third Minamata Disease (May 1973) drew public attention to the problems of Minamata Disease. There ensued a sudden increase in the number of applications for official certification. The certification process, conducted by the local government and the Certification Council, became clogged with excessive workload and unable to function properly. As a result, many applicants found themselves disqualified for certification. These applicants filed complaint after complaint about defective mass examinations, delayed decisions or unjustifiable rejections. They appealed to law-court or organised direct negotiations with the authorities concerned, demanding all the time that all applications should be accepted as soon as possible. They won all the cases at court, but neither the Environment Agency nor the Kumamoto prefectural government would accept the court decisions and appealed to higher courts. Thus, the certification system, in effect, has made a "great contribution" toward the reduction of officially certified patients. Disappointed with and in distrust of the government at large, the patients faced round to Chisso again, the primary source of harm and responsibility.

THE CERTIFICATION SYSTEM

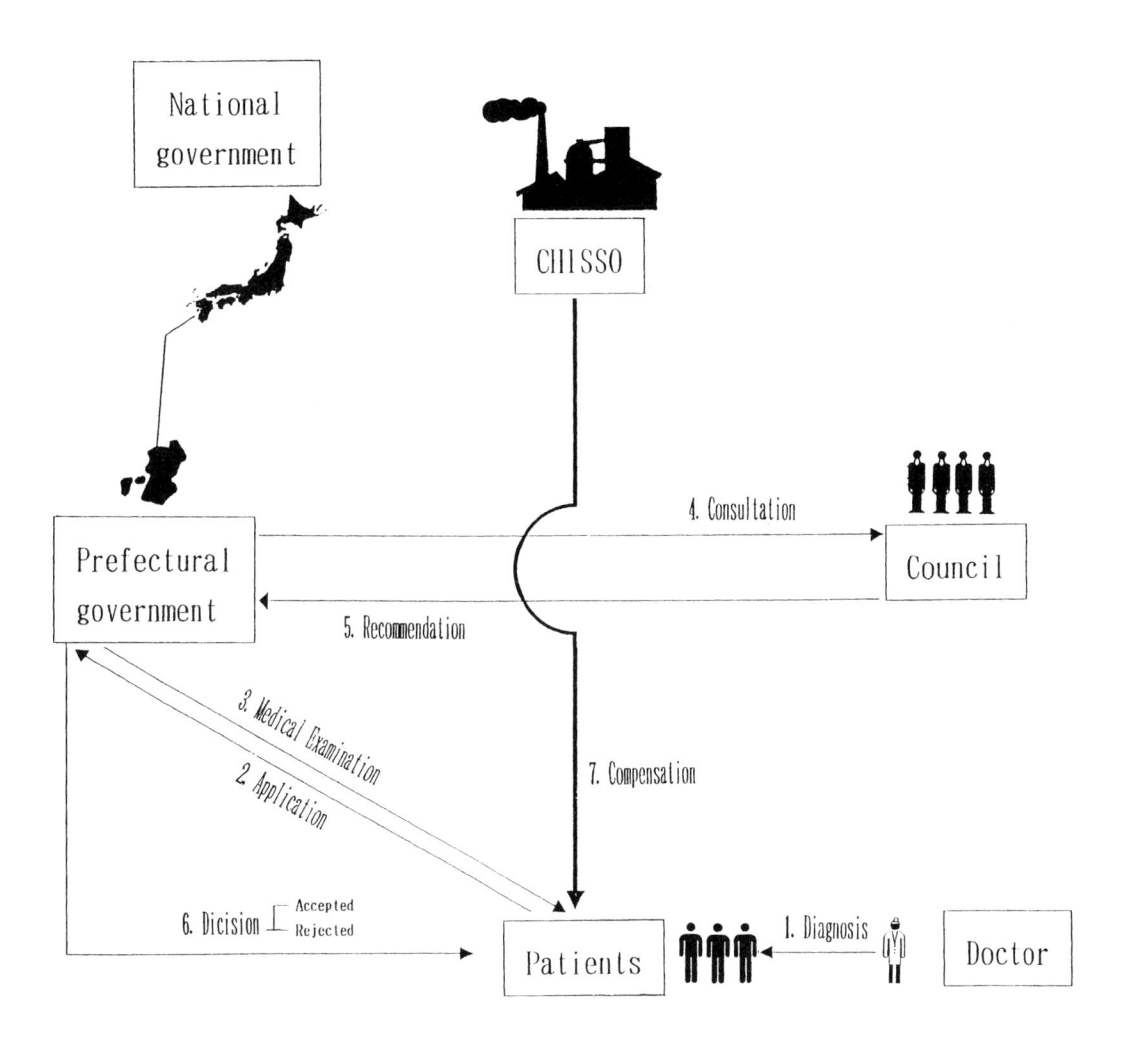

Minamata Disease patients must be "certified" by the government in order to get compensation from Chisso. Some of the qualifications stipulated for application are five-years' residence in the contaminated area on the Shiranui Sea and the acquisition of Minamata Disease symptoms. Qualified applicants submit their application, together with a medical certificate, to the Governor of their prefecture. The prefectural authorities arrange for the applicants to be examined; the medical reports are sent to the Certification Council made up of doctors. On the basis of the Council's recommendations, the Governor makes his decisions for or against applications. A great many questions, however, being asked of the certification system as it actually operates, in the light of the provisions of the Pollution Relief Fund Act (1971) and the current tight corner in which uncertified Minamata Disease patients find themselves.

CONS OUTWEIGH PROS IN THE APPLICATION FOR OFFICIAL CERTIFICATION

Surveyed by Sadao Togashi
Sadami Maruyama
(University of Kumamoto)1981

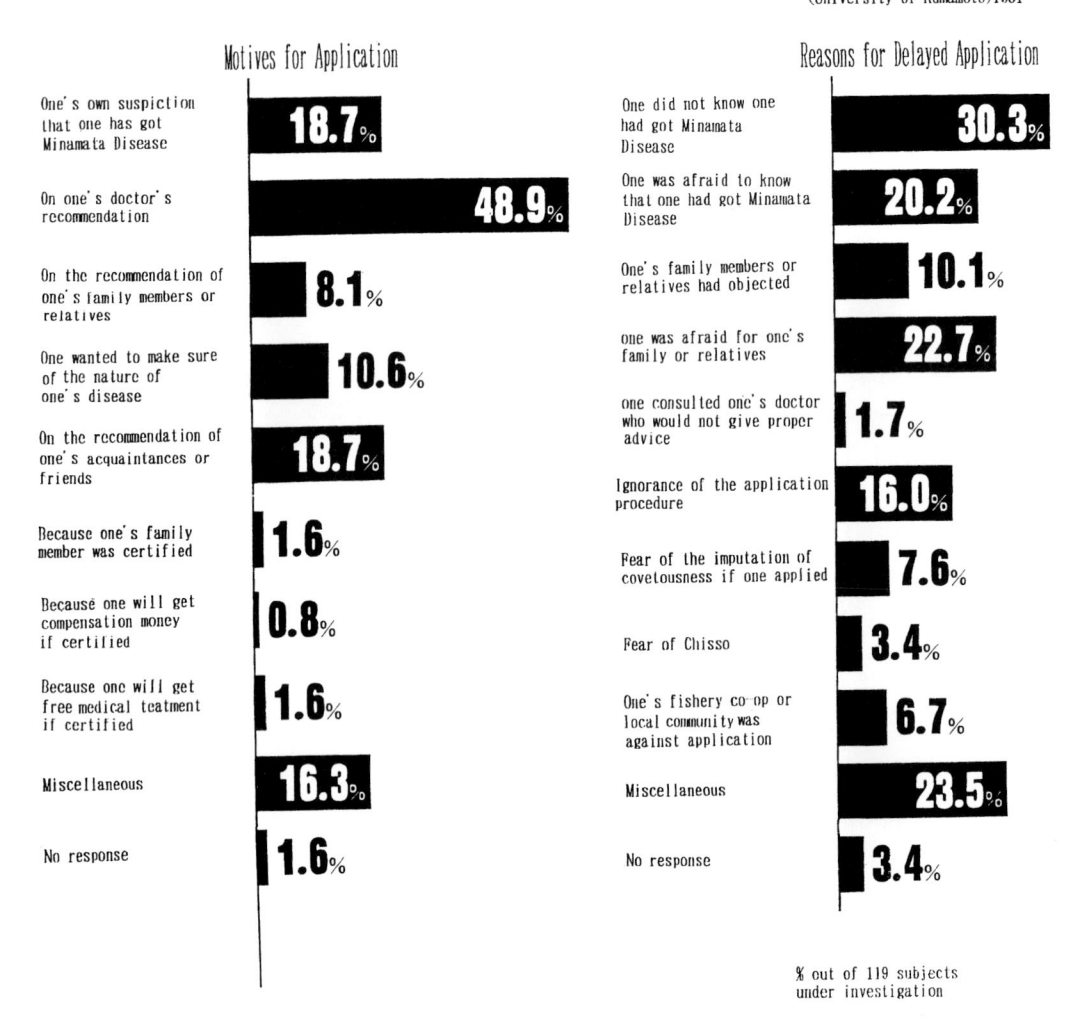

Motives for Application

Motive	%
One's own suspicion that one has got Minamata Disease	18.7%
On one's doctor's recommendation	48.9%
On the recommendation of one's family members or relatives	8.1%
One wanted to make sure of the nature of one's disease	10.6%
On the recommendation of one's acquaintances or friends	18.7%
Because one's family member was certified	1.6%
Because one will get compensation money if certified	0.8%
Because one will get free medical treatment if certified	1.6%
Miscellaneous	16.3%
No response	1.6%

Reasons for Delayed Application

Reason	%
One did not know one had got Minamata Disease	30.3%
One was afraid to know that one had got Minamata Disease	20.2%
One's family members or relatives had objected	10.1%
one was afraid for one's family or relatives	22.7%
one consulted one's doctor who would not give proper advice	1.7%
Ignorance of the application procedure	16.0%
Fear of the imputation of covetousness if one applied	7.6%
Fear of Chisso	3.4%
One's fishery co-op or local community was against application	6.7%
Miscellaneous	23.5%
No response	3.4%

% out of 119 subjects under investigation

It takes one a lot of courage simply to decide to apply. Many are deterred by fear and anxiety. Local people might say that "I won't marry a Minamata Disease patient or his family member" or "I didn't know you want money so much"——though Chisso will not do anything for one, however serious one's condition may get, unless one applies. Worse still, neither the national nor prefectural government has done anything in the way of public relations activities as to application procedure. Many victims say, "I did not know I had got Minamata Disease", even though they knew they had been eating fish.

APPLICATIONS REJECTED ONE AFTER ANOTHER

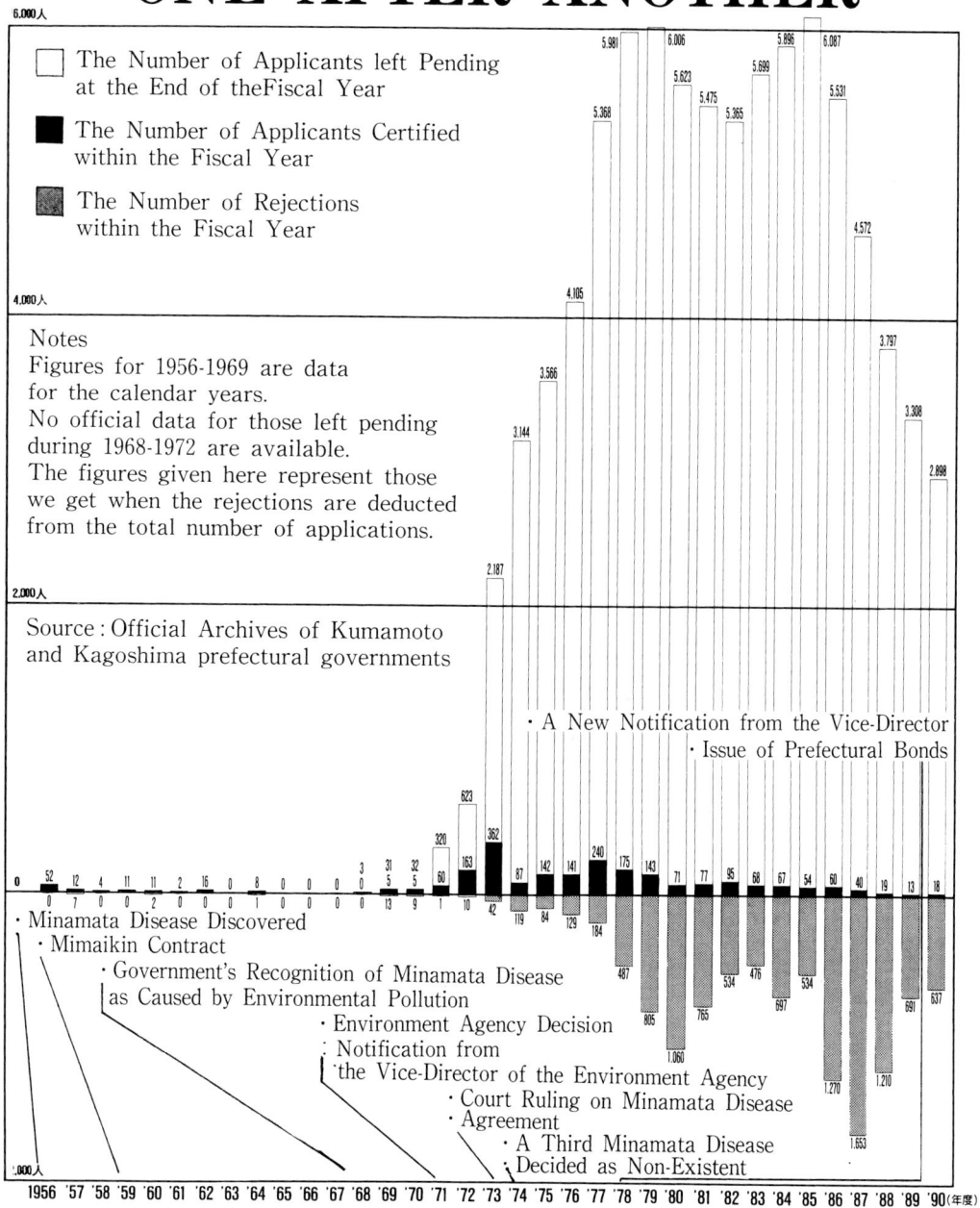

☐ The Number of Applicants left Pending at the End of the Fiscal Year

■ The Number of Applicants Certified within the Fiscal Year

▨ The Number of Rejections within the Fiscal Year

Notes
Figures for 1956-1969 are data for the calendar years.
No official data for those left pending during 1968-1972 are available.
The figures given here represent those we get when the rejections are deducted from the total number of applications.

Source: Official Archives of Kumamoto and Kagoshima prefectural governments

· A New Notification from the Vice-Director
· Issue of Prefectural Bonds
· Minamata Disease Discovered
· Mimaikin Contract
· Government's Recognition of Minamata Disease as Caused by Environmental Pollution
· Environment Agency Decision
· Notification from the Vice-Director of the Environment Agency
· Court Ruling on Minamata Disease
· Agreement
· A Third Minamata Disease Decided as Non-Existent

It may be said, with a fair degree of justice, that the certification system for Minamata Disease is intended, and, indeed, applied, to determine who is eligible for Chisso compensation instead of providing a system of criteria by which to judge who is a Minamata Disease patient. In other words, it is not too much to say that the system is something invented to protect the interests of Chisso. The original "criteria" have undergone frequent and radical revisions as applied by the national government (i.e. the Environment Agency), with the unfortunate result that, since 1973, a large proportion of applications submitted has met summary dismissal. There has remained a long queue of unaccepted patients in need of immediate relief; they are left out in the cold

THE NUMBER OF CERTIFIED PATIENTS

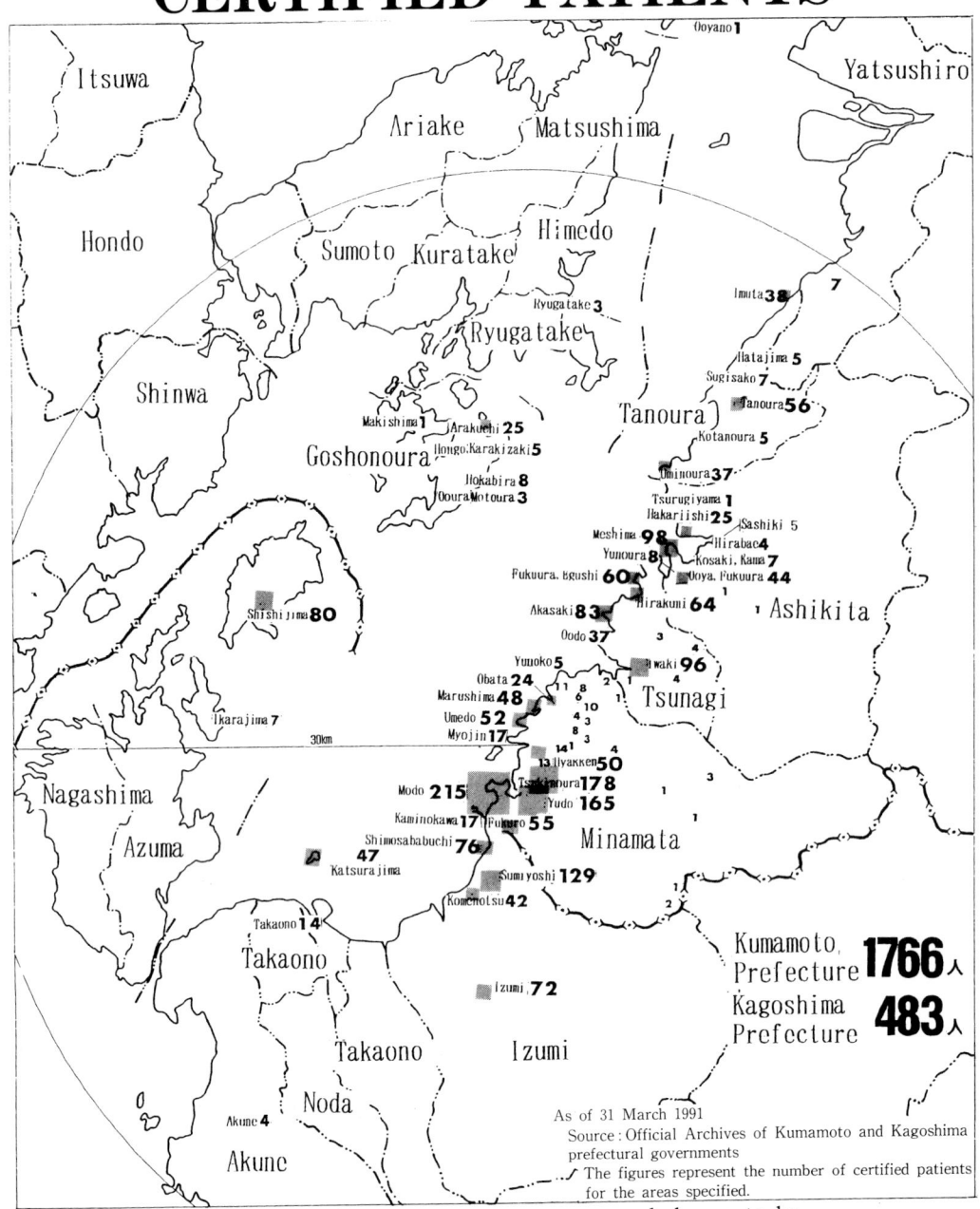

Ooyano 1
Itsuwa
Yatsushiro
Ariake Matsushima
Hondo
Sumoto Kuratake
Himedo
Ryugatake 3
Ryugatake
Imuta 38 7
Shinwa
Tanoura
Hatajima 5
Sugisako 7
Tanoura 56
Makishima 1 Arakuchi 25
Goshonoura Hongo,Karakizaki 5
Kotanoura 5
Uminoura 37
Hokabira 8
Tsurugiyama 1
Ooura,Motoura 3
Ikariishi 25 Sashiki 5
Meshima 9 8 Hirabae 4
Yunoura 8 Kosaki, Kama 7
Fukuura, Egushi 60 Ooya, Fukuura 44
Akasaki 83 Hirakumi 64
Shishijima 80
Oodo 37 Ashikita
Yunoko 5 Iwaki 96
Obata 24
Marushima 48 Tsunagi
Umedo 52
Ikarajima 7
Myojin 17
30km
Hyakken 50
Modo 215 Tsukinoura 178
Nagashima
Kaminokawa 17 Fukuro 55 Yudo 165
Azuma
Shimosahabuchi 76 Minamata
Katsurajima 47
Sumiyoshi 129
Komenotsu 42
Takaono 14
Takaono
Izumi 72
Kumamoto Prefecture **1766**人
Kagoshima Prefecture **483**人
Takaono
Noda Izumi
Akune 4
Akune

As of 31 March 1991
Source: Official Archives of Kumamoto and Kagoshima prefectural governments
The figures represent the number of certified patients for the areas specified.

Initially, at the time when organo-mercury compounds began to be discharged into the sea, nearly 300,000 people used to live on the Shiranui Sea. It is estimated, therefore, that tens of thousands of local residents were exposed to health hazards and suffered health damage of one kind or another, whether it was slight or serious. Only a handful of them have, so far, been certified and found eligible for compensation. Nobody knows, and nobody will know, how many more patients have got Minamata Disease and died without knowing why they were to die.

4
NOW——

WHAT SHOULD WE DO AND WHAT CAN WE DO?

THE PLIGHT OF UNCERTIFIED PATIENTS

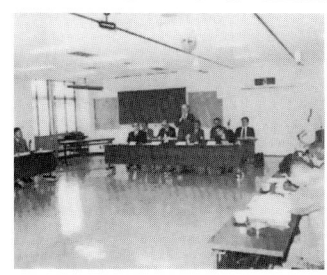

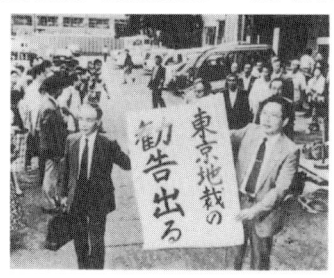

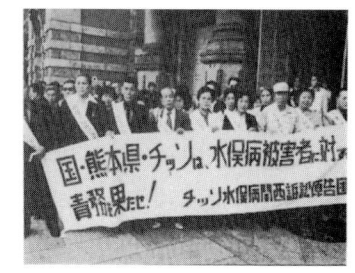

1   2   3

1. Members of the Group of Minamata Disease Patients for Negotiations with Chisso (now re-organised as the Association of Minamata Disease Patients with a membership of about 400) sat down in front of the Chisso premises, Minamata, in the autumn of 1988, and demanded compensation from Chisso. This sit-down tactics, which lasted for as long as half a year, was rewarded with success when Chisso agreed to sit at the negotiation table. The direct negotiations are still going on, with some Liberal-Democratic MPs, the Governor of Kumamoto prefecture and the Mayor of Minamata to mediate and witness their transactions.
2. About 1,900 uncertified patients, including those of the Society of Minamata Disease Victims, filed law suits at the district courts of Kumamoto, Tokyo, Kyoto and Fukuoka, demanding that the national government, the local government of Kumamoto prefecture, Chisso and its subsidiary companies should pay compensation. Their unflagging efforts were rewarded, in the autumn of 1990, with the court rulings in favour of the patients' request to the effect that those accused should agree to a friendly settlement. Such is the situation to date that the plaintiffs' counsel is engaged on consultations with the defendants except for the national government in an attempt to reach a reconciliatory settlement.
3. In the autumn of 1982, an independent group of about 70 patients, who had emigrated from the coastal area of the Shiranui Sea to the Kansai district and applied for official certification, went to law against the national government, the local government of Kumamoto and Chisso, asking for damages. Legal proceedings are still going on at the district court of Osaka. The patients are looking forward to winning their case.

The compensation agreement was signed in 1973 and Chisso was compelled to pay damages to officially certified patients. Unfortunately, it turned out that the local government was not so prompt and cooperative in their certification procedures as was hoped for. Those patients who found their applications dismissed or left pending were obliged to resort to a variety of tactics such as law-suits, direct negotiations or sit-downs, demanding a quick and positive settlement of as many applicants as was possible. The government, both at national and local levels, however, was adamant in their position: they were committed to protecting Chisso and would not accept the presence of an enormous number of patients in need of relief. Disappointed with the certification system and distressed at the imminent prospect of a crippled and helpless old age, many of the uncertified patients have now opted for a less hard line of discussions and reconciliation with the government, national and local, and Chisso. The only hope for them now is "immediate relief while we are alive".

THE PATIENTS ARE GETTING OLD

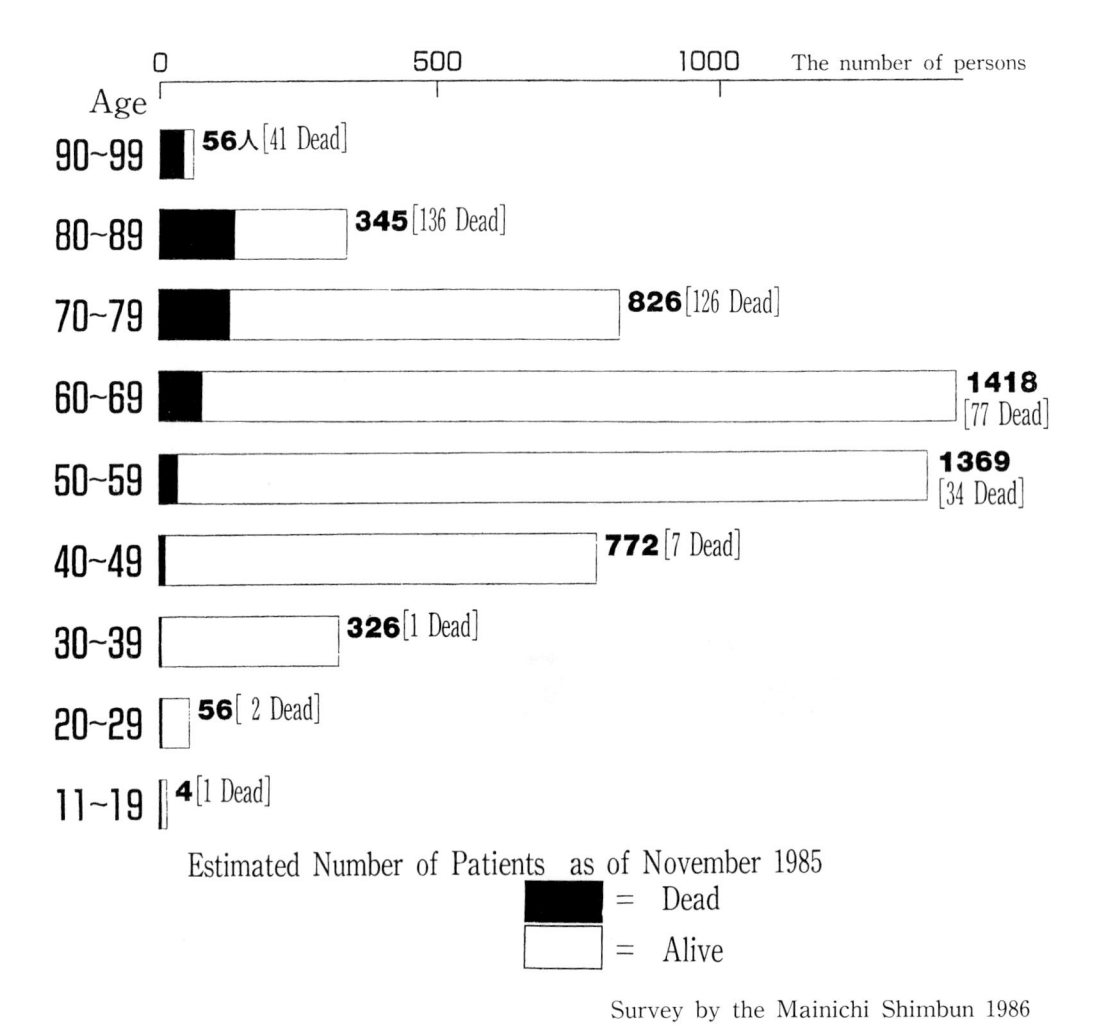

Age	Number	Dead
90~99	56	[41 Dead]
80~89	345	[136 Dead]
70~79	826	[126 Dead]
60~69	1418	[77 Dead]
50~59	1369	[34 Dead]
40~49	772	[7 Dead]
30~39	326	[1 Dead]
20~29	56	[2 Dead]
11~19	4	[1 Dead]

Estimated Number of Patients as of November 1985

■ = Dead
□ = Alive

Survey by the Mainichi Shimbun 1986

The older a patient becomes, the worse his symptoms grow. The average age of applicants now stands at around 60. An increasing number of young people, who have not yet applied for official certification, say that they also have Minamata Disease symptoms. Many of the patients who did apply have had their applications left in the balance for more than 10 years, whereas most of those few who were fortunate enough to get their applications accepted were certified after their post-mortem inspection. The patients are unanimous in complaining, "Should we wait until we are dead?"

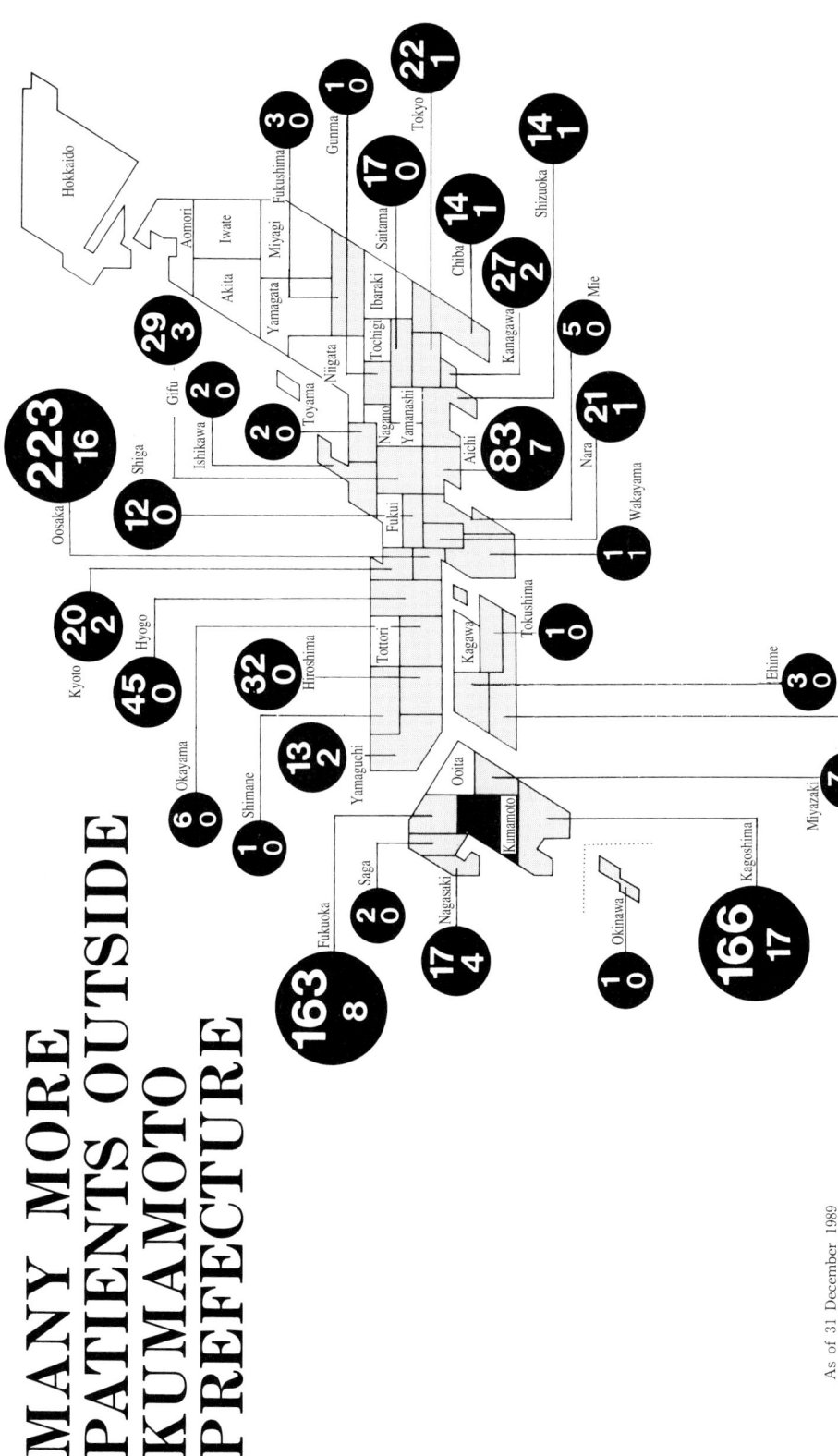

MANY MORE PATIENTS OUTSIDE KUMAMOTO PREFECTURE

As of 31 December 1989

The upper figure in each circle reprsents the total number of applicants and the lower one stands for the number of certified patients.

Prefecture	Applicants	Certified
Hokkaido	—	—
Aomori	—	—
Iwate	—	—
Miyagi	3	0
Akita	—	—
Yamagata	—	—
Fukushima	1	0
Niigata	29	3
Tochigi	—	—
Ibaraki	17	0
Gunma	1	0
Saitama	14	1
Tokyo	22	1
Chiba	27	2
Kanagawa	14	1
Shizuoka	14	1
Toyama	2	0
Ishikawa	2	0
Gifu	—	—
Nagano	—	—
Yamanashi	—	—
Aichi	83	7
Mie	5	0
Nara	21	1
Wakayama	1	1
Fukui	—	—
Shiga	12	0
Oosaka	223	16
Kyoto	20	2
Hyogo	45	0
Tottori	—	—
Okayama	6	0
Hiroshima	32	0
Shimane	1	0
Yamaguchi	13	2
Kagawa	1	0
Tokushima	—	—
Ehime	3	0
Kochi	5	0
Fukuoka	163	8
Saga	2	0
Nagasaki	17	4
Ooita	—	—
Kumamoto	—	—
Miyazaki	7	0
Kagoshima	166	17
Okinawa	1	0

It is unfortunate that Minamata Disease is not yet understood in its true light. That is partly why "outside patients" find themselves in a variety of distressful situations.

* Access to proper medical services is difficult because local doctors are not familiar with the symtoms of Minamata Disease.
* Local doctors' unwillingness to follow the proper procedure compels the patient to pay medical expenses out of his pocket.
* Some patients are discriminated against because their neighbours believe that "Minamata Disease" is contagious.
* The patient is afraid to declare that he is a Minamata Disease patient, so he is often labelled as a "lazy fellow" when he says he is unwell.
* The patient has few people in his or her neighbourhood whom he or she can trust and rely on.
* Some patients are not aware that they are afflicted by Minamata Disease because they have little chance to learn about the disease.

It is estimated that nearly 300,000 people have lived on the Shiranui Sea since Chisso started dumping their mercury-contaminated effluents into the sea. Quite a few of them, who used to make their living by fishing, left the sea and emigrated to cities to look for employment. Some of them who went to Tokyo, Kyoto and Osaka, had their first signs of Minamata Disease or found their symptoms getting worse after emigration. They united themselves into local groups of patients and appealed to the law for redemption and relief. They are still active now. But incomprehension and misunderstanding, which prevail in their neighbourhoods and in their local governments, have added to the anguish and distress that they and their family members have been suffering from.

SEDIMENTS DREDGED OUT AND THE BAY FILLED IN

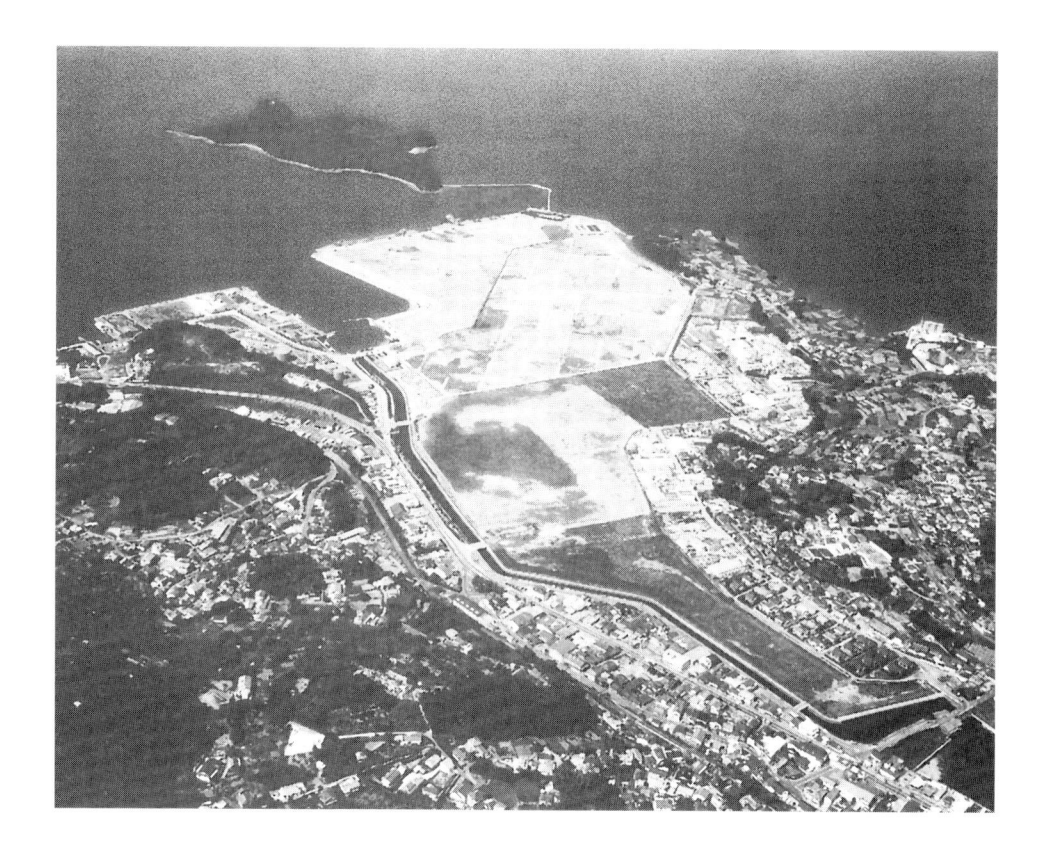

   Mercury-contaminated sediments are found all over Minamata Bay, but only a small portion of them with a mercury content of more than 25ppm has been dredged out of the sea which in turn has been filled in. The land thus reclaimed covers an area of 520,000m² ——a large new addition to the land area of Minamata City at the cost of more than 40,000,000,000 yen. Some Minamata citizens were afraid that the whole project might casue additional contamination and took legal action against it. They lost their case because it was ruled that "there is no possibility of additional contamination as the operations are well organised and well supervised". The rest of the sedements left at the sea bottom still continues to contaminate the Shiranui Sea and all the fish in it.

MERCURY WAS IN USE ALL OVER JAPAN

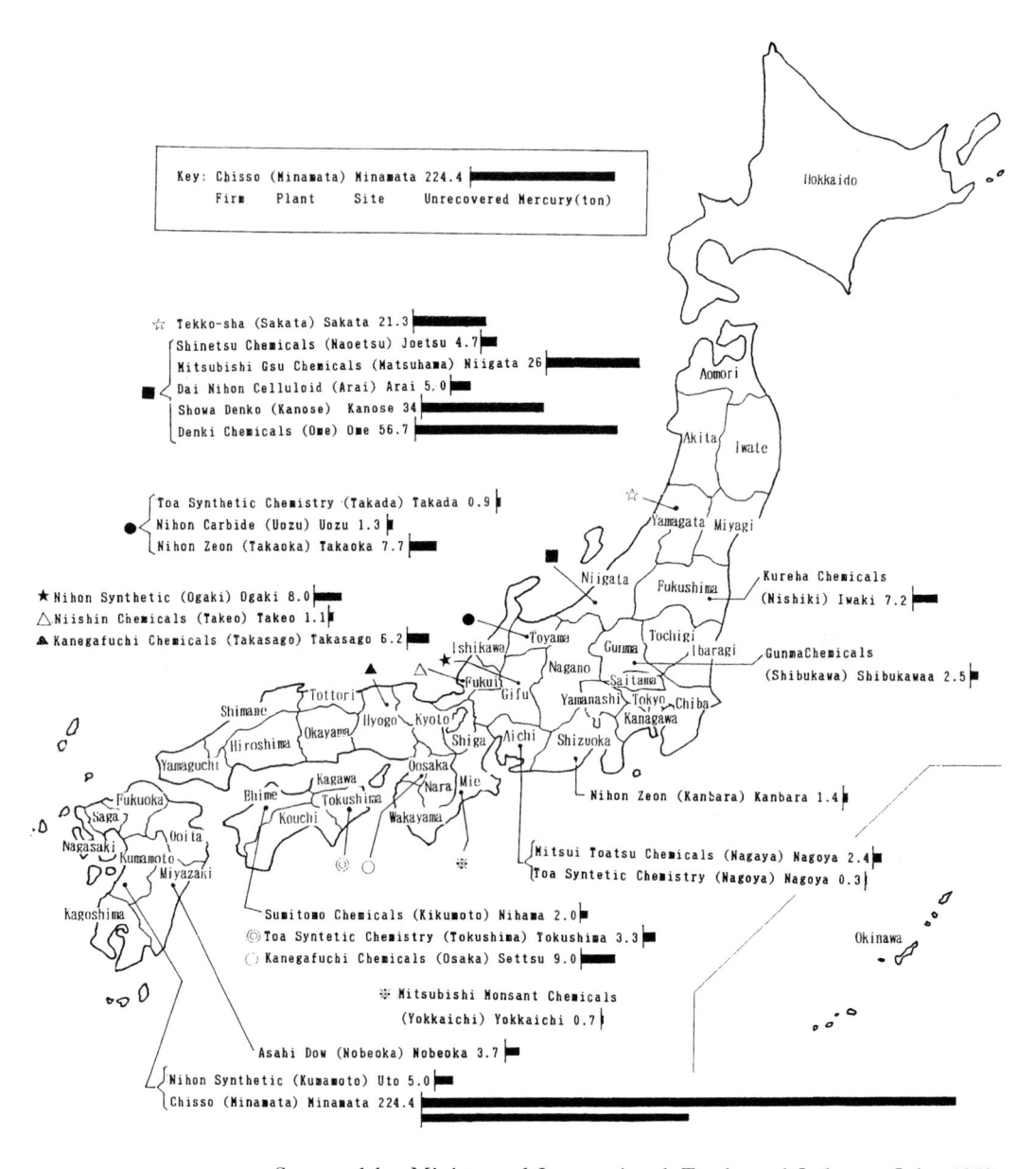

Key: Chisso (Minamata) Minamata 224.4
Firm   Plant   Site   Unrecovered Mercury(ton)

☆ Tekko-sha (Sakata) Sakata 21.3
Shinetsu Chemicals (Naoetsu) Joetsu 4.7
Mitsubishi Gsu Chemicals (Matsuhama) Niigata 26
■ Dai Nihon Celluloid (Arai) Arai 5.0
Showa Denko (Kanose) Kanose 34
Denki Chemicals (Ome) Ome 56.7

Toa Synthetic Chemistry (Takada) Takada 0.9
● Nihon Carbide (Uozu) Uozu 1.3
Nihon Zeon (Takaoka) Takaoka 7.7

★ Nihon Synthetic (Ogaki) Ogaki 8.0
△ Niishin Chemicals (Takeo) Takeo 1.1
▲ Kanegafuchi Chemicals (Takasago) Takasago 6.2

Kureha Chemicals (Nishiki) Iwaki 7.2

Gunma Chemicals (Shibukawa) Shibukawaa 2.5

Nihon Zeon (Kanbara) Kanbara 1.4

Mitsui Toatsu Chemicals (Nagaya) Nagoya 2.4
Toa Synetic Chemistry (Nagoya) Nagoya 0.3

Sumitomo Chemicals (Kikumoto) Nihama 2.0
◎ Toa Synetic Chemistry (Tokushima) Tokushima 3.3
○ Kanegafuchi Chemicals (Osaka) Settsu 9.0

❋ Mitsubishi Monsant Chemicals (Yokkaichi) Yokkaichi 0.7

Asahi Dow (Nobeoka) Nobeoka 3.7
Nihon Synthetic (Kumamoto) Uto 5.0
Chisso (Minamata) Minamata 224.4

Surveyed by Ministry of International Trade and Industry July, 1973

Just like Chisso, many chemical plants used mercury and discharged it into the sea. It will remain undiminished for dozens of years. Agricultural chemicals containing mercury were also in use for a while and those mercury compounds also flowed into the sea.

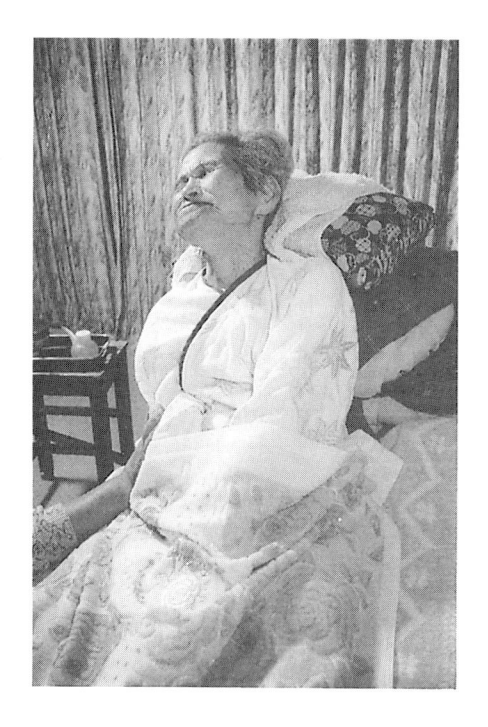

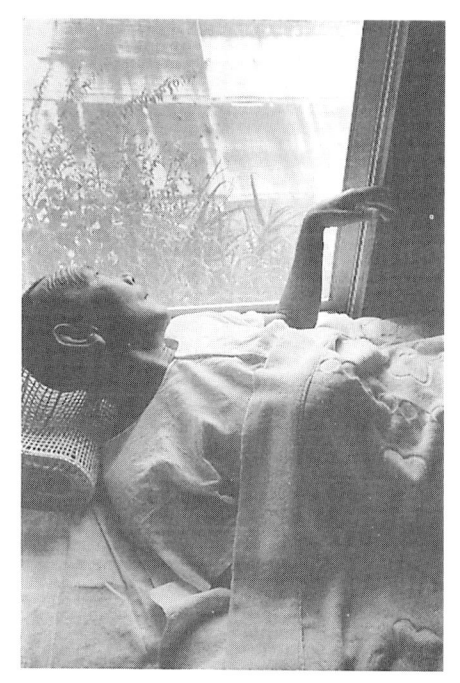

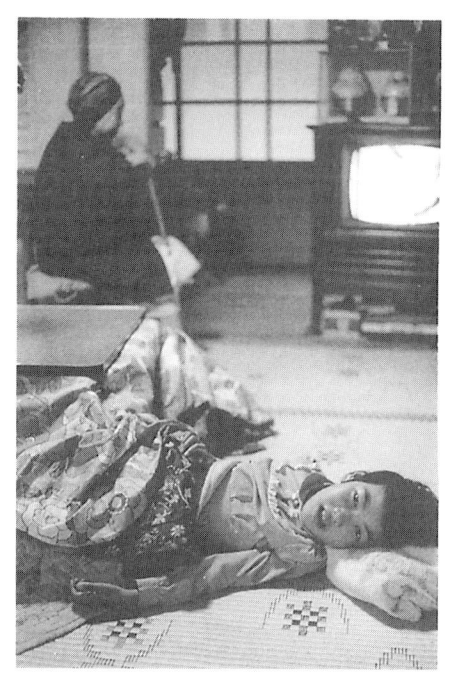

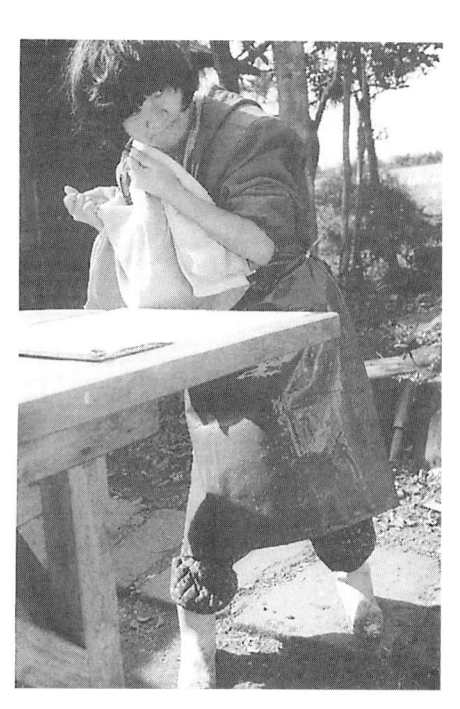

Photographed by Akutagawa Jin 1979—1991

PATIENTS IN PROTEST AGAINST THE IMPUTATION OF "FAKE PATIENTS"

Photographed by Akutagawa Jin 1979

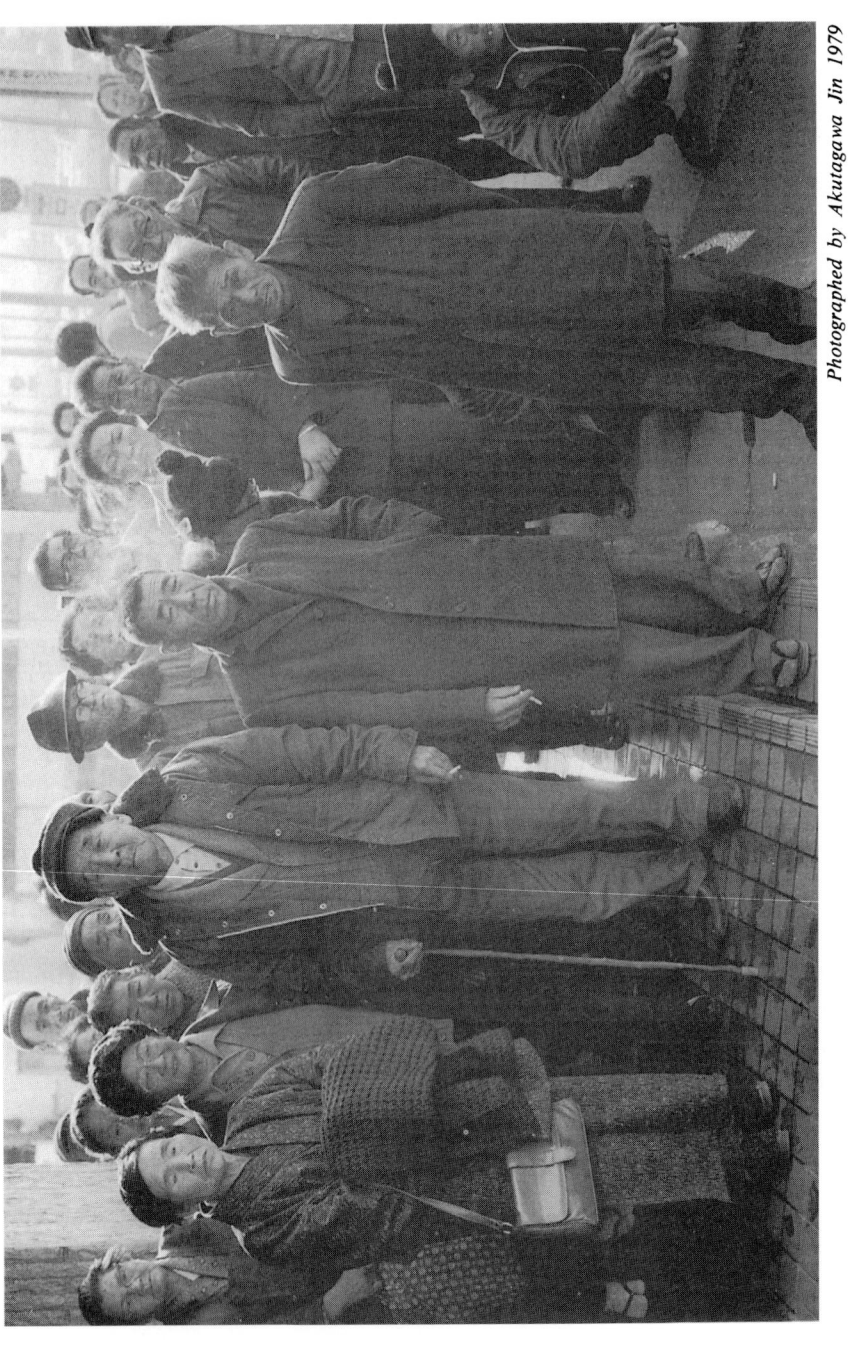

MINAMATA DISEASE IS NOT OVER YET

The case of Minamata Disease is still left unsolved more than 30 years after its initial discovery. Certified patients are denied access to as much adequate medical care or livelihood relief as they deserve whereas those still uncertified are left in the cold. There are many other problems yet to be solved. Chisso and the government, however, are waiting for all the patients to die, deliberately blind to the long-standing weight of anguish and sufferings under which the victims have been groaning. The most important lesson to be learned from Minamata Disease is, in the light of the enormous breadth and depth of its harm, that "it is not a disease but it represents the irredeemable destruction of life and nature". This is not a local incident which happened to take place at a particular place (i.e. on the Shiranui Sea) but it is both symbolic and symptomatic of a world-wide disaster: our world is being overrun with more pollution problems than ca be counted. Accidents will happen at nuclear power stations which are being constructed one after another. We could be overwhelmed at any moment by massive amounts of nuclear wastes and radioactive fallout. Our earth is being covered with poisonous substances and radioactivity. What is there that we can ever leave to our children and their children?

MINAMATA DISEASE CENTRE SOSHISHA

Why Minamata Disease Centre Soshisha was founded:
The purpose of this Foundation is to help Minamata Disease victims and their relatives to solve problems in the general conduct of their daily life and to conduct research work on Minamata Disease.
Founded ; 7 April 1974
Managing Director : Hiroki Iwamoto

What Soshisha aims at:
Soshisha, situated on a hill-side, overlooks the calm waters of the Shiranui Sea. Also visible is a small graveyard nestled among the surrounding hills. That is where victims of Minamata Disease are buried: they did not know what killed them. They were killed by Chisso and the government.

Soshisha, as well as the Museum, stands on the side of the Minamata Disease victims and inhabitants on the Shiranui Sea who have had their life and livelihood destroyed. We are with them in an everlasting effort to bring to light the facts of Minamata Disease and to investigate its implications. Contemporary society is generally geared to the idea of " convenience and plenty ", so that nuclear power stations, food additives, or the breakdown of school discipline are nothing but news of passing interest instead of being consciousness-awakening problems.

Soshisha and the Museum have neither power nor influence to call society to account or to mobilise public opinion. We are determined, however, to continue to " record and communicate " until the day comes when we have no Minamata Disease problem. We have decided that it is our ' will ' and our job to get closer and ever closer to what and how Minamata Disease victims feel.

Services
Soshisha offers services listed below.
1. Services for those who wish to study or research Minamata Disease at Minamata including:
   1-1 : Overnight accomodation for up to 20 members at 1,000 yen per person per night. Reservation is required. No meals are served.
   1-2 : Study sessions and guided tours which can be arranged as appropriate.
   1-3 : Information service at our data room. Prior arrangements are required.
2. One week summer course, organised by Soshisha and called Minamata Action School, which is open to those who wish to observe and study Minamata Disease on the spot. Information is available on request.
3. *Gonzui* (Marine Catfish), bulletin of Soshisha, is issued 6 times a year. This bi-monthly pamphlet is primarily centred on the significant implications of the tragedy of Minamata Disease for our conduct of life in the present and future. Annual subscription is welcome at 2,000 yen.

Minamata Disease Museum

The Minamata Disease Museum was founded on 26 September 1988 in the premises of Soshisha on a hill overlooking the Shiranui Sea.

More than 35 years have passed since the official discovery in 1956 of Minamata Disease, but full details of the damage done to life, health and the environment are yet to come to light. Minamata Disease is not over yet. It can not be over. On the contrary, the tragic consequences of mercury poisoning and contamination are everywhere in evidence and they challenge every one of us to cope with them. We are required to look Minamata Disease in the face, to reflect on its problems and implications in the historical context of Japan's modernisation and idustrialisation and to sort them out so that both the present and future generations will learn lessons from them.

The Minamata Disease Museum is not intented to exhibit relics from the past, but to collect fresh information and materials, to conduct research work on the various related problem of Minamata Disease and to let the public know the results of our activities. We expect our members and visitors to offer constructive comments and responses, which, we are sure, will help us to be more creative and efficient in our approaches and strategies. Ours is a dynamic institution.

Exhibits: The Museum is divided into four sections.
　　　　[The Shiranui Sea —— A Beautiful Sea and A Bountiful Life]
　　　　[Minamata Disease —— Chisso's Crime]
　　　　[A Long Struggle —— Thirty Years of Victimization and Sufferings]
　　　　[Now —— What Should We Do and What Can We Do?]

The exhibits include nearly 100 photographs and illustration panels, wooden boats, fishing tackle, Chisso's products and the ' cat shed ' where Chisso medical staff conducted experiments on cats.

Open: 9.00——17.00
Closed: Mondays (except when they fall on public holidays) and during
　　　　New Year holidays
Admission: 300 yen for high school children and adults
　　　　　　200 yen for elementary and junior high school pupils
For Sale and Hire: books and video-tapes on Minamata Disease are on sale
　　　　　　　　　at the shop and video films are for hire from the office.
School tours: group tours can be arranged with the office.
Mobile exhibitions: exhibition panels, Chisso's products and fishing tackle are
　　　　　　　　　　available for hire. Mobile exhibitions can be arranged with
　　　　　　　　　　the office.

Sustaining Members are Welcome:

Both Soshisha and the Minamata Disease Museum are funded and supported by sustaining members. Our principle now is that we should work together with anyone who will not only take an interest in our affairs but also take an active part in them so that our joint concern wtih Minamata Disease may help us in working out a viable ideology and strategy to cope with worldwide problems.

Your wisdom and cooperation are welcome. Please join us as a sustaining member.
　　＊Annual Fee: 10,000 yen (one unit)
　　＊Postal Transfer Number: Minamata Disease Centre Soshisah, Kumamoto
　　　　　　　　　　　　　　9-25341
　　＊Members' benefits: A special gift on application and renewal of membership
　　　　　　　　　　　　A free delivery of Gonzui 6 times a year
　　　　　　　　　　　　Free admission to the Museum and free accomodation at
　　　　　　　　　　　　Soshisha
　　　　　　　　　　　　Discounts on video-tapes and films on sale and for hire

＊Full details are available from the office.

Map of Soshisha premises:

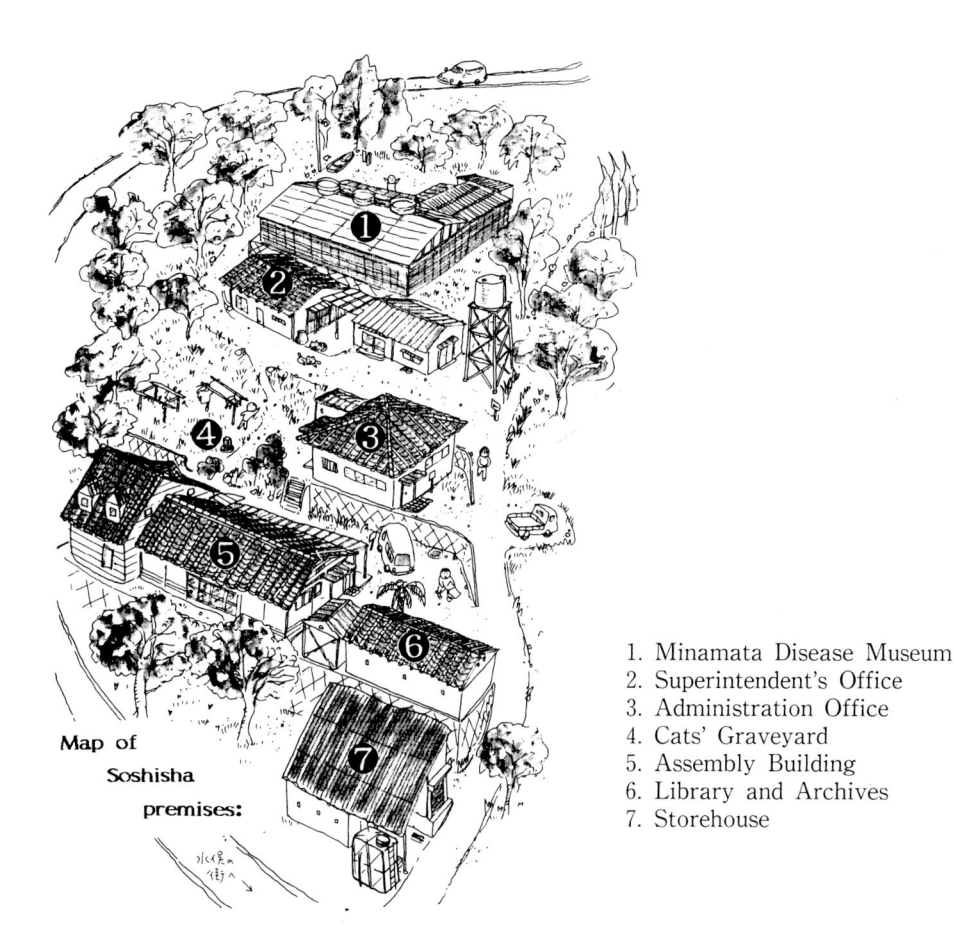

1. Minamata Disease Museum
2. Superintendent's Office
3. Administration Office
4. Cats' Graveyard
5. Assembly Building
6. Library and Archives
7. Storehouse

Transport: Approaches to Soshisha and the Minamata Disease Museum

Railways: Minamata Station on the JR Kagoshima Trunk Line
Buses: There are two bus services available from Minamata Railway Station. One is run by Nangoku Bus Co.. Buses bound for Izumi stop at Yudo. The Museum is a 15 minutes' walk from the bus stop. Sanko buses bound for Modo stop at Detsuki. It takes 12 minutes to walk to the Museum.
Taxis: It is a 10 minutes' taxi ride from the railway station.
Walking: The pedestrian may cover the distance in an hour or more.

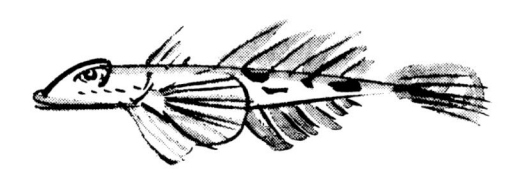

Summary History of the Minamata Disease Case

1908 Chisso's plant was built at Minamata village
1932 Acetalydehyde plant (where mercury was used) came into operation
1949 A remarkble decrease in the fish catch at Minamata Bay
1953 A "Cat Dancing Disease" was witnessed at Modo and Detsuki
1956 Official discovery of Minamata Disease
1957 Friendly Association of Minamata Disease Patients and their Relatives was organised
1959 Mimaikin contract
1961 Congenital Minamata Disease cases were discovered
1963 Minamata Disease was discovered in Niigata
1966 Cessation of mercury-polluted effluents from Chisso
1968 National government's official recognition of Minamata Disease as a disease caused by environmental pollution
1969 First law suit at Kumamoto District Court
1971 Independent negotiations started with sit-ins in front of Chisso's head office
1972 Victims made an appeal at the UN Conference on the Human Environment
1973 Kumamoto District Court ruling. Plaintiff won. A third Minamata Disease was reported
1974 Minamata Disease Centre Soshisha was founded. Council of Applicants for Official Certification was organised.
1975 "Fake patient comment" from Sugimura, member of Kumamoto Prefectural Assembly
1977 Appeal was filed for the cessation of sludge disposal operations at Minamata Bay.
A dividing net was set in Minamata Bay.
Minamata Action School was started
1980 Appeal for the cessation of sludge disposal was turned down. The third law suit was filed
1982 Minamta Disease patients in the Kansai district appealed to the law
1986 The 30th anniversary of the official discovery of Minamata Disease. Asian People's Convention was held
1988 The Minamata Disease Museum was founded
1989 The Federation of Minamata Disease Patients was organised.
All directors of Soshisha resigned due to the so-called "Sweet Summer Orange" incident
1990 Anti-pollution operations at Minamata Bay were declared to be finished

Foundation
Minamata Disease Centre Soshinsha
Minamata Disease Museum
〒867-0034 Fukuro, Minamata, Kumamoto Prefecture
Tel: 0966-63-5800 (81-966-63-5800)
Fax: 0966-63-5808 (81-966-63-5808)
E-mail info@soshinsha.org

絵で見る
水 俣 病

財団法人　水俣病センター相思社
水俣病歴史考証館

絵で見る水俣病
目次

はじめに　93

1　不知火海──豊かな海と暮し

　不知火海は波静かで小さな海　97
　海と人びと　98
　水俣近辺の「えびすさん」　99
　打瀬網　100
　巾着網　101
　「昔しゃなんでんかんでん作っとったもん」　102
　「はんのうはんぎょ海と畑半分こ」　103
　ボラ籠　104
　不知火海のおもな漁法　105

2　水俣病──チッソの犯罪

　チッソ　109
　戦前の主なチッソ製品　110
　身の回りのチッソ製品　111
　朝鮮チッソ興南工場　112
　チッソ水俣工場　113
　水銀の流出とチッソの加害行為　114

アセトアルデヒドを作るため水銀が使われた　115
メチル水銀は工場から海へ　116
魚のすみかが失われた　117
チッソ城下町・水俣　118
水銀は魚介類をへて人びとへ　119
健康被害　120
水銀が神経細胞を破壊する　121
母体を通して水銀は胎児へ　122
全身に症状が　123
書字障害　124
苦痛は生活の中で拡大する　125
汚染は不知火海全域に広がった　126
不知火海全域から水俣病申請患者が　127
20万人以上の被害者が裾野に拡がっている　129
被害は病苦を越えて　130
患者はどのような治療をしているのか　131
多様な被害　132
政治家たちの患者非難　133
こんな言葉が投げつけられた　134

3 闘い―被害者の30年

　　原因究明期　137

　　まず猫が狂い死にをした―1954年　138

　　水俣病が発見された―1956年　139

　　汚染魚は放置された―1957年　140

　　漁民は立ち上った―1959年　141

　　患者たちはやっと立ち上った―1959年　142

　　患者をだましたチッソ契約―1959年　143

　　患者運動高揚期　144

　　水俣病裁判判決　145

　　協定書・補償の現状　146

　　社長との直接交渉　147

　　自主交渉坐り込み　148

　　支援活動　149

　　認定制度への闘い　150

　　認定・補償の仕組み　151

　　認定申請そのものが困難　152

　　申請しても切りすてられる　153

　　これまでに認定された人びと　154

4　現在―私たちの課題

水俣湾のヘドロ処理　157
水俣湾の仕切網と魚介類の現状　158
仕切網の変遷　159
水俣湾内の魚介類の水銀値と仕切網　160
チッソ貸付資金のしくみ　161
チッソの経営状況　162
未認定患者の現状　163
政府解決案に伴うチッソ支援などのしくみ　164
1994年7月11日水俣病関西訴訟の一審判決　165
行政にも責任がある　166
もやい直しの始まり　168
水俣病を問い続ける　169
水俣病の教訓を生かすために　170
財団法人　水俣病センター相思社　171

はじめに

　水俣病を英語で紹介する本をつくりました。ILLUSTRATED MINAMATA DISEASE（絵で見る水俣病）というタイトルで、主に水俣病歴史考証館の陳列パネルを使って説明しています。日本文も添えました。

　アマゾン流域の水銀中毒が危惧され、さまざまの微量毒性物質の、地球的規模での、堆積汚染が指摘されている現在、水俣病のもつ意味は重大になってきています。

　水俣病は戦争による被害でもなく、避けられなかった過失でもありません。企業の生産活動における、技術的制約から生じた不可避的な公害でもありません。公害とは「私企業並びに公企業の活動によって地域住民のこうむる人為的災害」と言えます。しかし一般的には「市民生活の役に立つ生産活動によって起きた害」と考えられており、万やむをえず人びとに害を与えてしまったが、それは仕方がない害であると考えられている節さえあります。

　水俣病の拡大は、承知のうえで、企業の利潤追求と、それを指導し追認し保護する国の方針によってなされたのです。そこには人びとの福祉を重んじ、環境を保護する姿勢はありませんでした。

　日本の戦後の復興と、西欧に追い付き追い越せという高度経済成長は、なるほど、国家が栄え企業が発展すれば、人びとの福祉は自動的に実現するという思想を土台にしていたかも知れません。そして貧しいがゆえに、多くの日本人がそのような思想やそれに基づく施策を支持したかもしれません。しかしその誤りは日本の人びとの現在の暮らしを見れば明らかです。何よりも水俣病に苦しむ人びとがその誤りを如実に体現し、告発しています。

　この本は、貧しさにあえぎ経済発展を切望し、日本が一つの手本になるのではないかと考えるアジア・アフリカ・南米諸国のすべての人びとに向けた、水俣からの切実なメッセージです。

　この本はマグサイサイ賞財団と千葉大学の南田正児先生のご協力なしには実現しませんでした。ここに深く感謝の意を表します。

不知火海──豊かな海と暮し 1

不知火海は波静かで小さな海

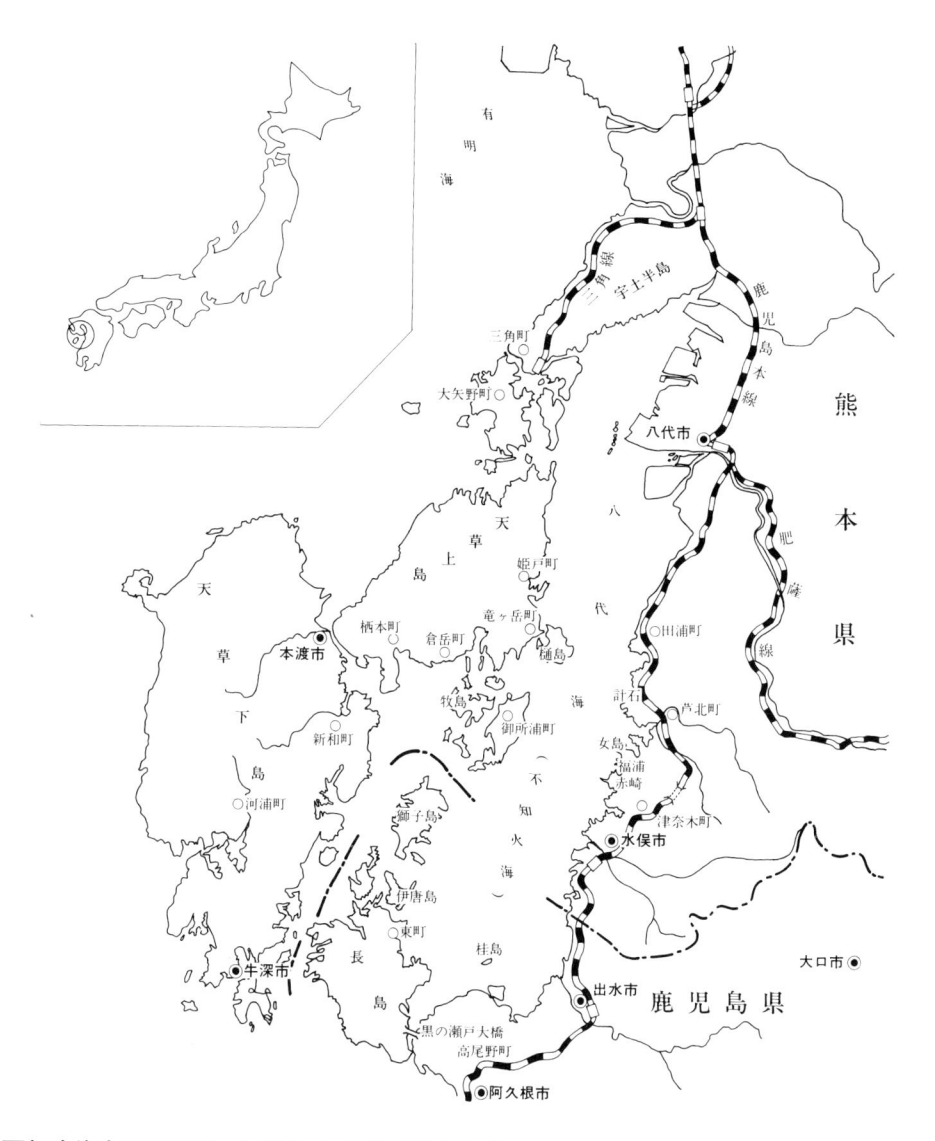

不知火海(八代海)は、九州本土と天草諸島によって囲まれた内海である。面積は約1,400km²(琵琶湖程度)で、東西6〜16km、南北70kmと細長く、水深は平均50mほどだが、干潮・満潮の差は4mもある。水俣を中心とした南部の地形は変化に富み、魚や貝の産卵する場所もいたる所にあって、たくさんの種類の生き物たちが暮している。

海と人びと

　水俣から見える不知火海は、鏡のような凪(なぎ)に照らされる対岸の天草の島々を映しだす。台風でもないかぎり、漁師は毎日のように手こぎ舟を沖へ出す。舟の上で、あるいは家族とともに、獲れたての魚と焼酎で舌つづみを打つ。ひと山越えた村々からも、潮の香りに誘われて、カキ打ち、ビナ拾いにやってくる。不知火海は、海辺の人びとをふところ深く包み込み、質素な中にも、豊かな自然の恵みのあるあたたかい暮しを与え続けてきた。

水俣近辺の「えびすさん」

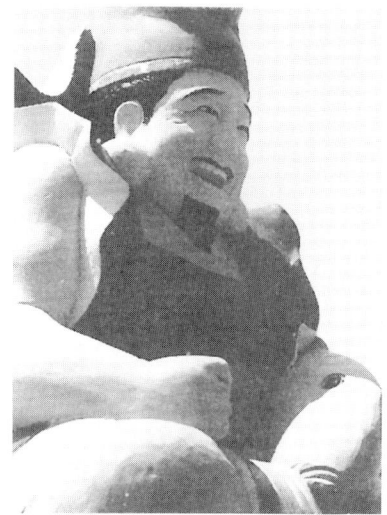

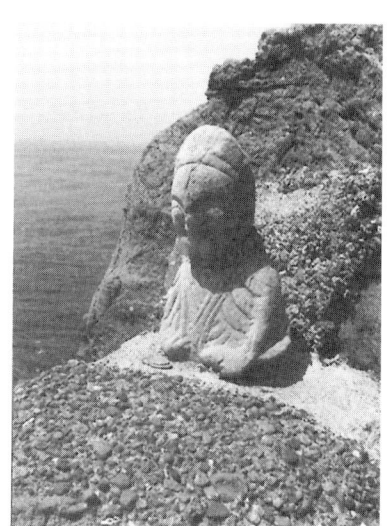

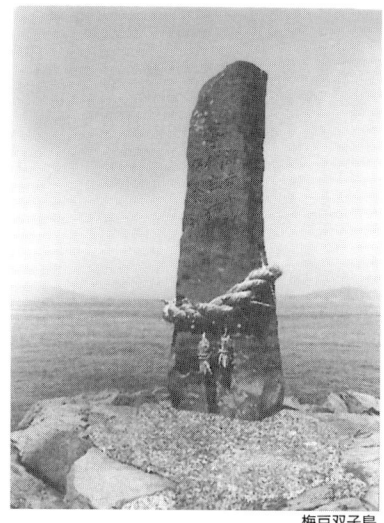

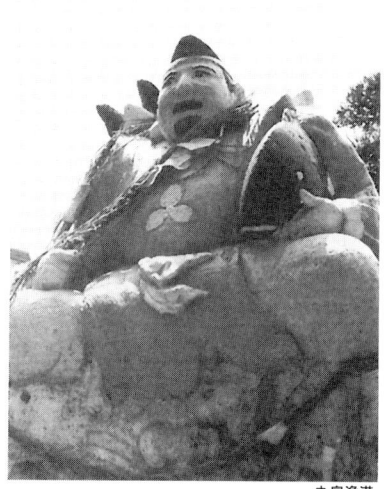

梅戸漁港

梅戸双子島

梅戸双子島

丸島漁港

撮影　芥川仁　1978年

この地方の漁師部落には必ずと言ってよいほど、えびすの石像がみられる。「えびす様」は魚をもたらしてくれる神として信仰され、年2回は漁を休んで祭りをした。海とともに生きる人々の、海に対する思いや畏の深さをあらわしている。

打三瀬網

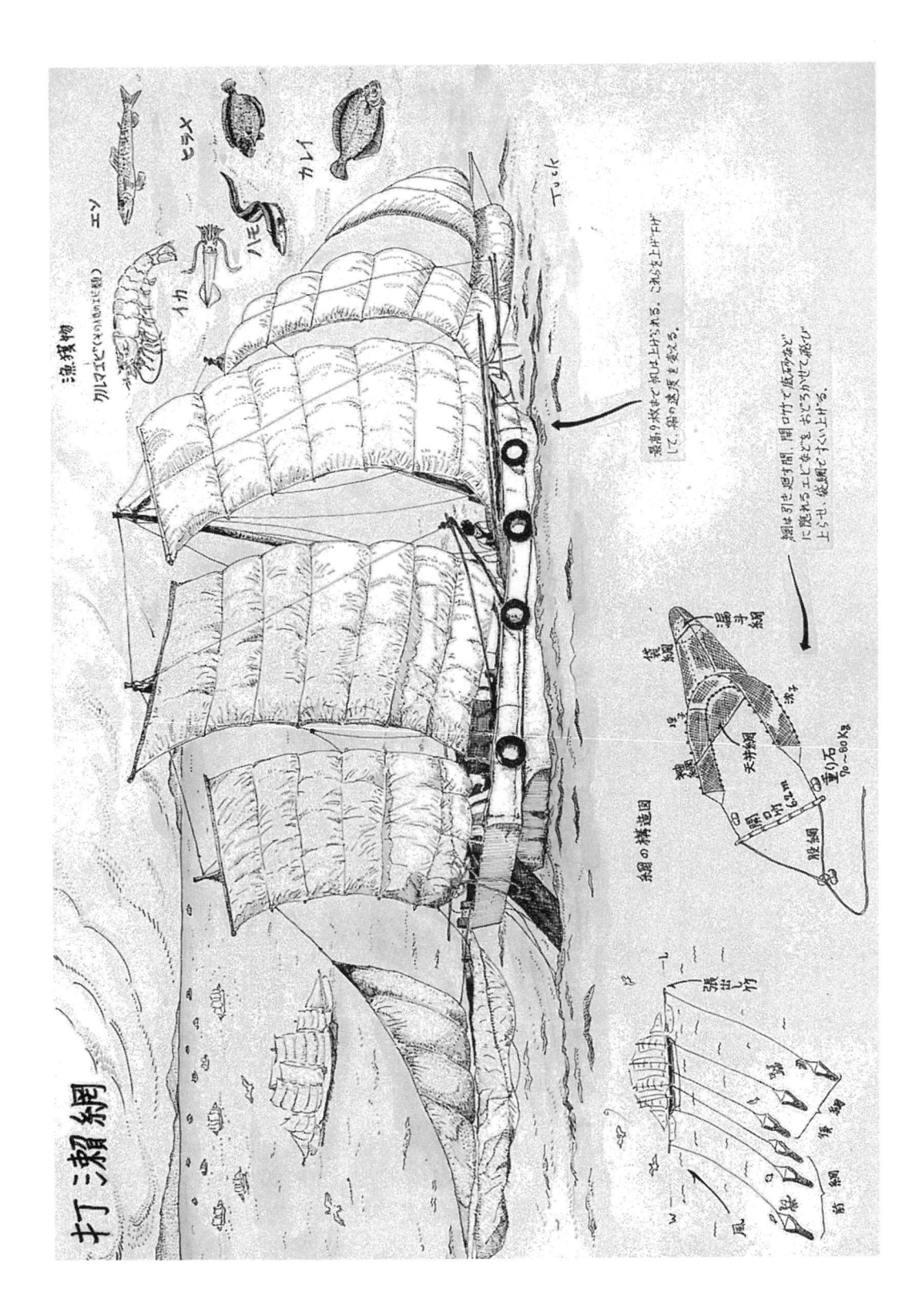

漁獲物
- クルマエビ(くもんぱ広を聞)
- エビ
- イカ
- ハモ
- カレイ
- ヒラメ

網は引き道す間、開口けで底砂など
に隠れたエビなどをおどろかせて浮び
上らせ、袋網でスくいとっていく。

最後9米まで手ぐりあげられ、これらを上げすげ
て、袋の魚を反を集える。

袋網の構造図
- 袋網
- 揚手網
- 親網
- 天井網
- 6.2m
- 股網
- 重り石 70〜80Kg

（風向き図）
- 張出し竹
- 天井網
- 股網
- 袋網
- 親網
- 風 W→

鯛網漁

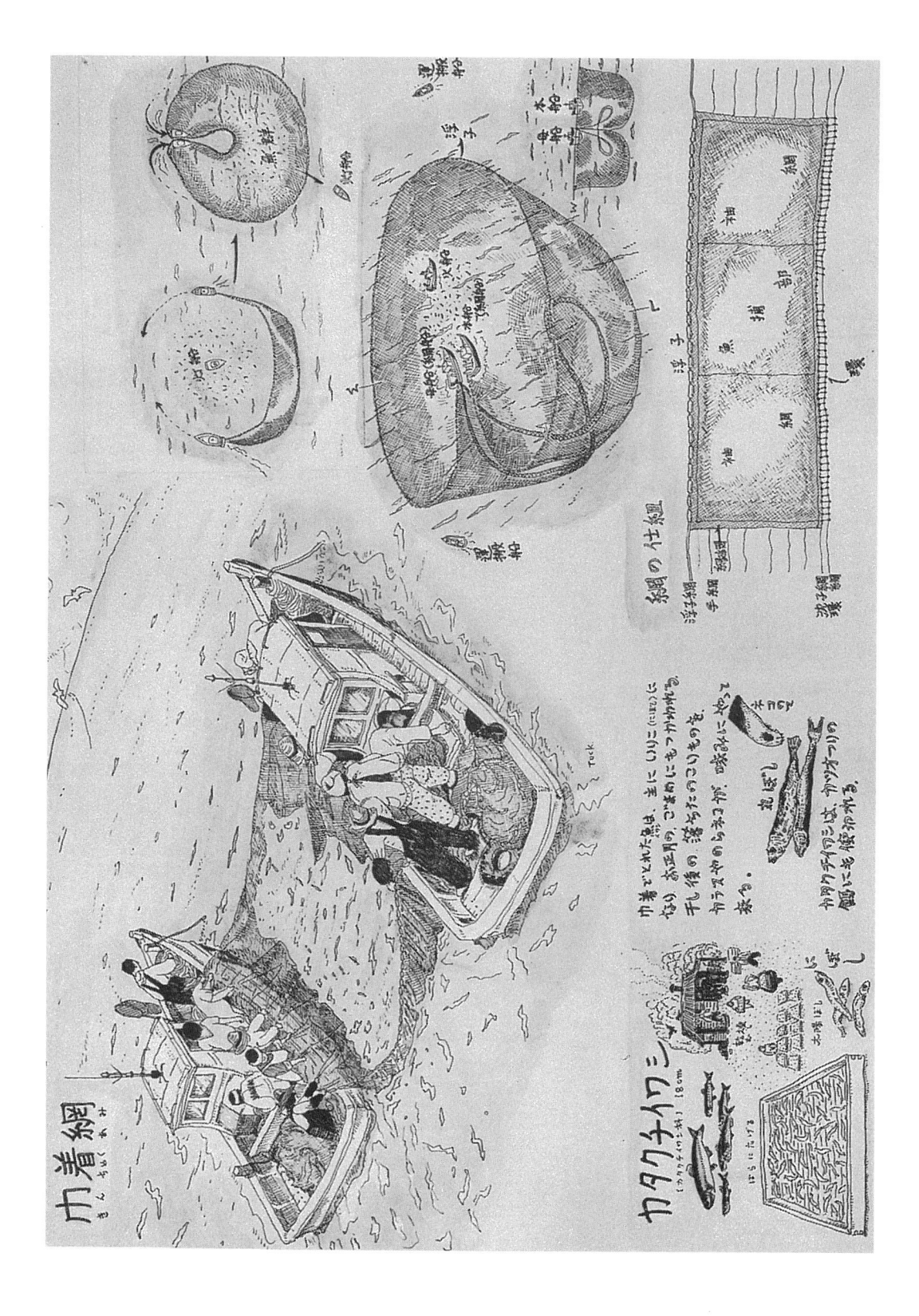

鯛網の仕組

カタクチイワシ

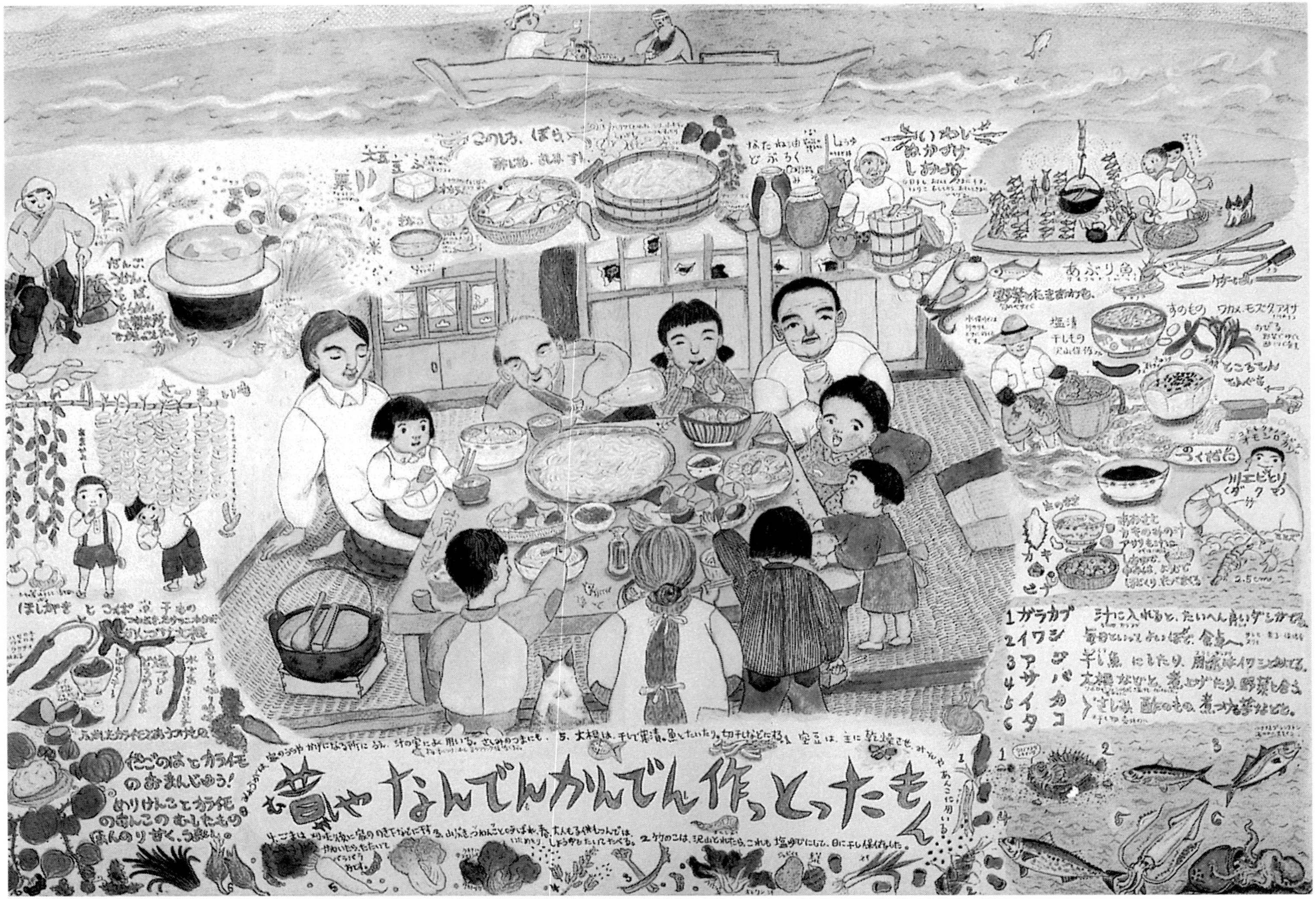

昔じゃ なんでんかんでん作っとったもん
1 ガラカブ
2 イワシ
3 アジ
4 サバ
5 イカ
6 タコ
汁に入れると、たいへん良いダシがでる。
干し魚 にしたり、
あぶり魚
すのもの
つくだに

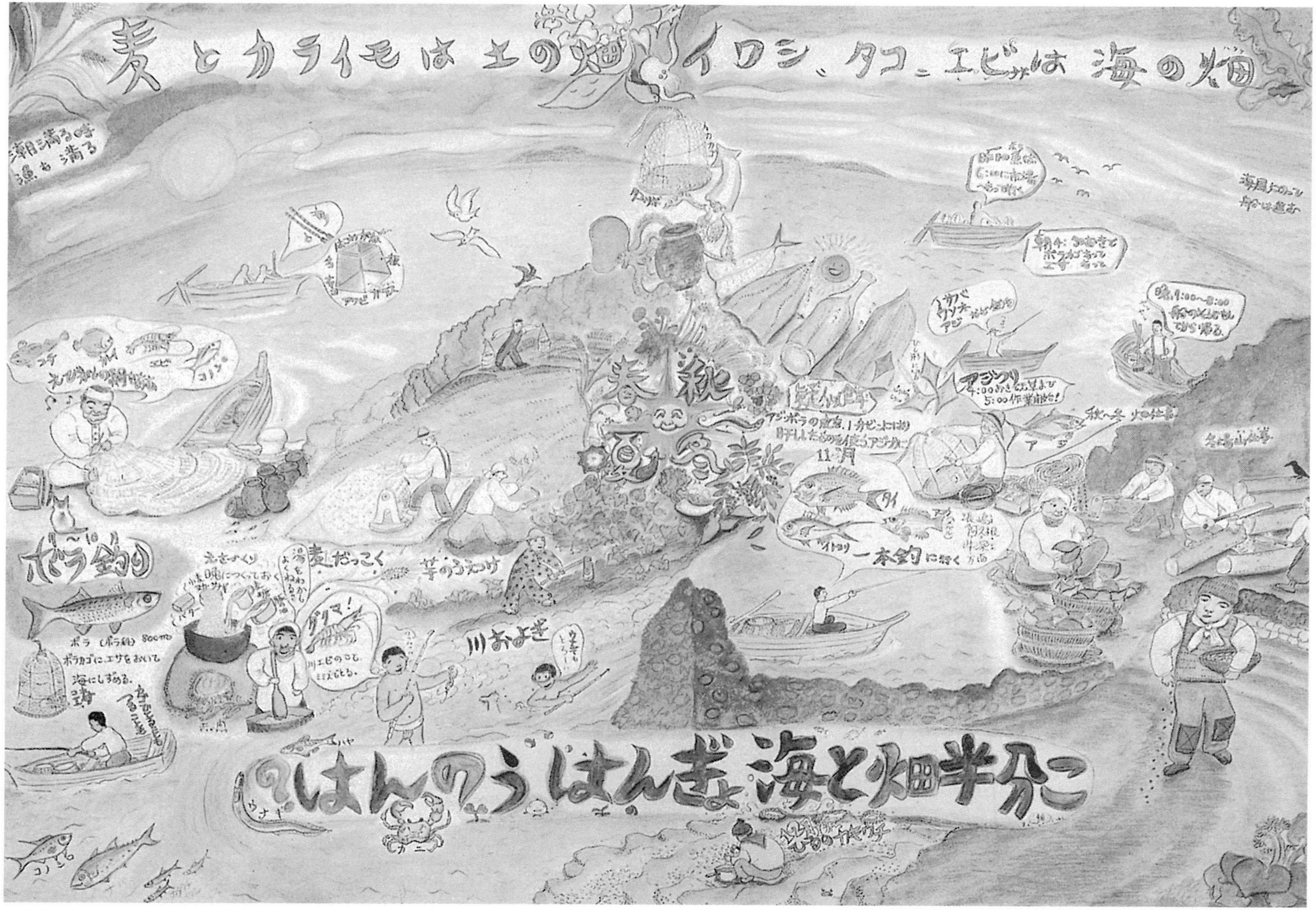
麦とカライモは土の畑 イワシ、タコ、エビは海の畑
潮満る時 魚も満る
ボラ釣り
麦だっこく
芋のうえつけ
川およぎ
一本釣に行く
春 秋 夏 冬
11月
はんのうはんぎょ 海と畑半分こ

ボラ竹籠

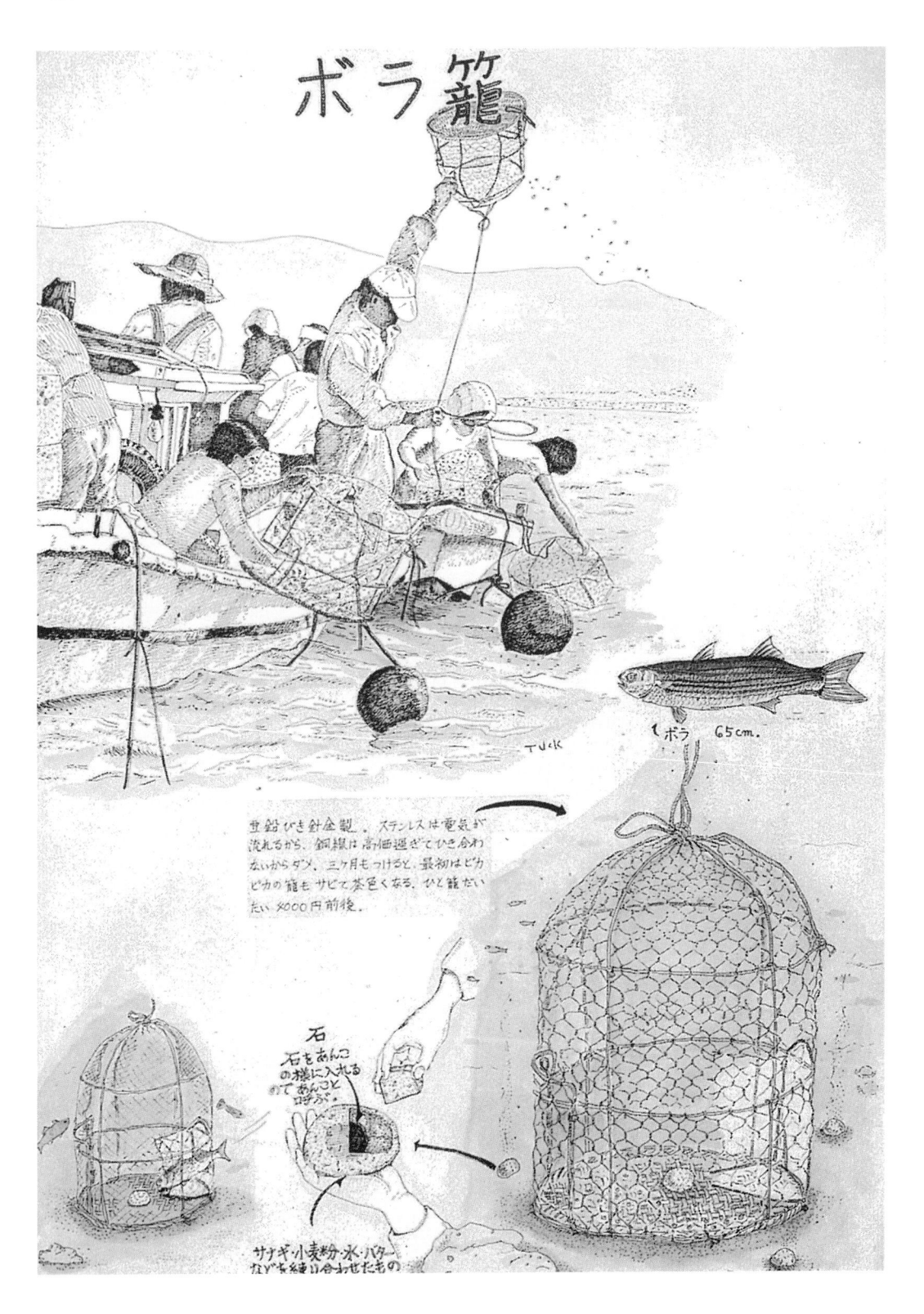

亜鉛びき針金製。ステンレスは電気が
流れるから、銅線は高価過ぎてひき合わ
ないからダメ、三ヶ月もつけると、最初はピカ
ピカの籠もサビて茶色くなる。ひと籠だい
たい4000円前後。

ボラ 65cm.

石
石をあんこ
の様に入れる
のであんごと
呼ぶ。

サナギ・小麦粉・水・バター
などを練り合わせたもの

不知火海のおもな漁法

手繰り網
小型機船底引き網の一種。エビ、カレイ、タコ、イカなどを比較的浅場で獲る。田浦でよく行なわれる。

えさびき網
小型機船底引き網の一種。釣りや延縄用のエサを獲る。現在ではタイの一本釣りに用いる生きエビ獲りに、御所浦で行なわれている。

貝けた網
小型機船底引き網の一種。

なまこけた網
小型機船底引き網の一種。

打瀬網
小型無動力船引き網の一種。漁場では動力を止め、風力で網を引く。現在では芦北郡の計石が主流。イセエビ、クルマエビ、イカ、ハモ、エソ、ヒラメなどを獲る。

巾着網
中型巻き網の一種。カタクチイワシをおもに、マイワシ、アジ、サバなども獲る。イワシは、イリコ製造とカツオ船の生きエサ用。現在は獅子島、天草東岸海域だけで行なわれている。

改良網（シロ網）
小型巻き網の一種。巾着網より小型で、これにかわって台頭。イリコ製造用、カタクチイワシも獲る。

吾智網
船は1槽、少人数で行なう。手繰り網と似ているが、船で網を引っ張らない。現在では不知火海の代表的な漁法で、タイ、グチ、ハモ、タチウオなどを獲る。

一本釣り
タイ、アジ、タコ、イサキ、フグ釣りなどが代表的。時期、場所、対象魚によって釣り方はさまざま。

鉾つき
おもに夜操業する。鉾で魚の頭をねらってつく。

タコ獲り
海岸で腰まで海につかり、箱メガネを使って鉾でタコをつく。

イワシ機船引き網
主にカタクチイワシ。イリコ製造用。

刺し網
古くからの漁法。潮流を遮断するように1〜3枚の網を入れ、魚を刺したり、網をからめたりして獲る漁法。エビ流し網、カニカシ網、クツゾコ刺し網などがある。

イカかご
かごを沈めて産卵にくるイカを獲る。

ボラかご
エサの入ったかごを沈めて誘い込む。

カニかご
エサの入ったかごを沈めて誘い込む。

タコつぼ
つぼを海底に沈めて捕らえる。

羽瀬（ハゼ）
定置網の一種。八代地先などの浅場で行なわれる独特の漁法。網の入口の周囲に1列に竹を刺し、魚を誘い込む。コチ、エビ、カレイなどを獲る。

地引き網
昭和の初めまで不知火海の代表的漁法。カタクチイワシをおもに狙う。むかしは部落総出で網を引いた。

延縄
ガラカブ延縄などが代表的。釣針を数10本糸にならべ、海にたらす。

カキ打ち
岩についているカキの殻を道具を使って割り、中の実を獲る。

ビナ獲り
潮の引いた浅瀬で岩についている巻貝を獲る。

不知火海を産卵場とする魚種は大変多く、その特色を生かしたさまざまな釣り、網、壺、籠などの漁法が古くから発達してきたが、不知火海の漁業を代表するのはイワシ漁である。古くは地引き網によって行われていたが、動力船が導入されるようになると巻き網漁（巾着網）が主力となる。これは人手をかなり必要とするため、この地域に網元、網子制度が確立した。しかし昭和30年代から40年代のイワシの不漁、給料制の導入、水俣病の発生などにより、経営が成り立たなくなる網元が増えた。その後はイワシ漁にかわって、少人数でできる吾智網漁や刺し網漁が圧倒的に多くなった。特に昭和40年頃より始まった養殖漁業の台頭は目ざましく、今日では不知火海の水揚げの半分以上を占めており、海の汚染などが深刻な問題となっている。

水俣病――チッソの犯罪 2

チッソ

チッソの創業は、1906(明治39)年、鹿児島に設立した電力会社「曽木電気株式会社」に始まる。その後、化学肥料の製造で飛躍的に業績を伸ばし、第一次世界大戦後には、朝鮮侵略によって、日本有数の総合化学会社にまで成長をとげた。主要工場のあった水俣では、チッソは「城主」として君臨し、社会・経済全般にわたって影響力を深めた。旧財閥に比べ、後進のチッソが急成長した鍵は、安全対策を欠いた、一貫した利潤追求第一主義にあった。

戦前の主なチッソ製品

1937(昭和12)年発行「日本窒素肥料事業大観」より

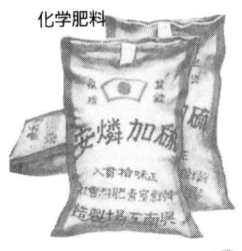

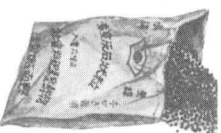

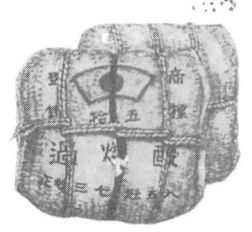

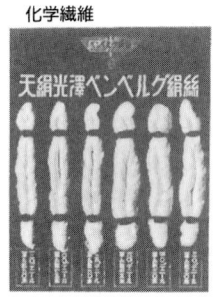

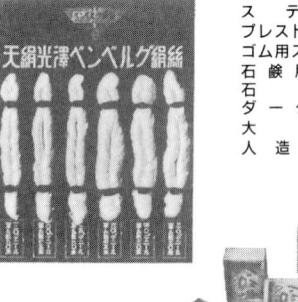

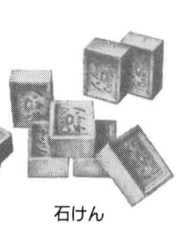

化学肥料

肥料
硫安
硫燐安
硫燐加安
石灰窒素
過燐酸石灰
調合肥料

工業薬品(工業材料)
アンモニア水
無水アンモニア
液体アンモニア
40度硝酸
98%硝酸
硝酸アンモニア
氷酢酸
無水酢酸
アセトアルデヒド
アカバイト
カミナリット
ミナロイド
ビニールアセテート
チッソロイド
硫酸
塩素
液体塩素
さらし粉
苛性ソーダ
ソーダ灰
塩化アンモン
亜硝酸ソーダ
珪フッ化ソーダ
硅酸ソーダ
蟻酸
硼酸
硫酸銅
ペンタエリスリット
無水塩化アルミニウム
エチレングリコール
旭味(化学調味料)
アミノ酸醤油

石炭工業
石炭
重油
揮発油
練炭
半成コークス
パラフィン
クレオソート
メタノール
ホルマリン
ヘキサメチレンテトラミン
アスファルト
ピッチ
車軸油
合成タンニン
チッソライト板
チッソライトコンパウンド
チッソライト成型品

その他
酸素
窒素
アルゴン
炭素電極
溶解カーボン
カーボンブラック
マグネシウムクリンカー
マグネシウム金属
マグネシウム合金
銑鉄
水銀
合成宝石

人造絹糸(化学繊維)
ベンベルグ絹糸
ヴィスコース糸
ステープルファイバー
酢酸人絹

火薬
膠質ダイナマイト
硝安ダイナマイト
硝安爆薬
黒色鉱山火薬
導火線用粉火薬
緩燃導火線
工業用雷管
電気雷管

油脂
硬化油
グリセリン
脂肪酸
ステロール
プレストステアリン
ゴム用ステアリン酸
石鹸用脂肪酸
ダークオイル
大豆油
人造バター

工業薬品

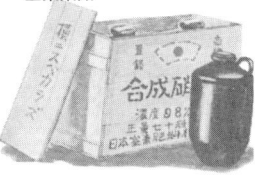

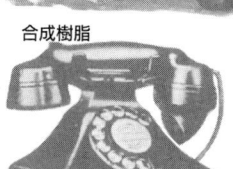

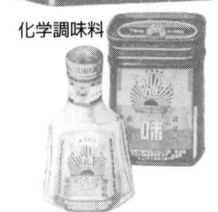

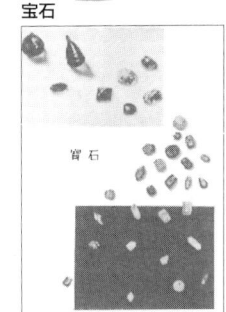

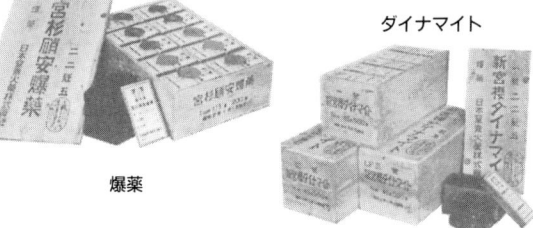

合成樹脂

化学調味料

宝石

化学繊維

石けん

爆薬

ダイナマイト

チッソは「総合化学会社」として、石けん・化学調味料などの日用品から、酢酸・硫酸などの工業用品、火薬など軍需品まで作っていた。"チッソの歴史は日本化学工業の歴史"といわれ、業界のパイオニアとして、その名は世界にも知られていた。

身の回りのチッソ製品

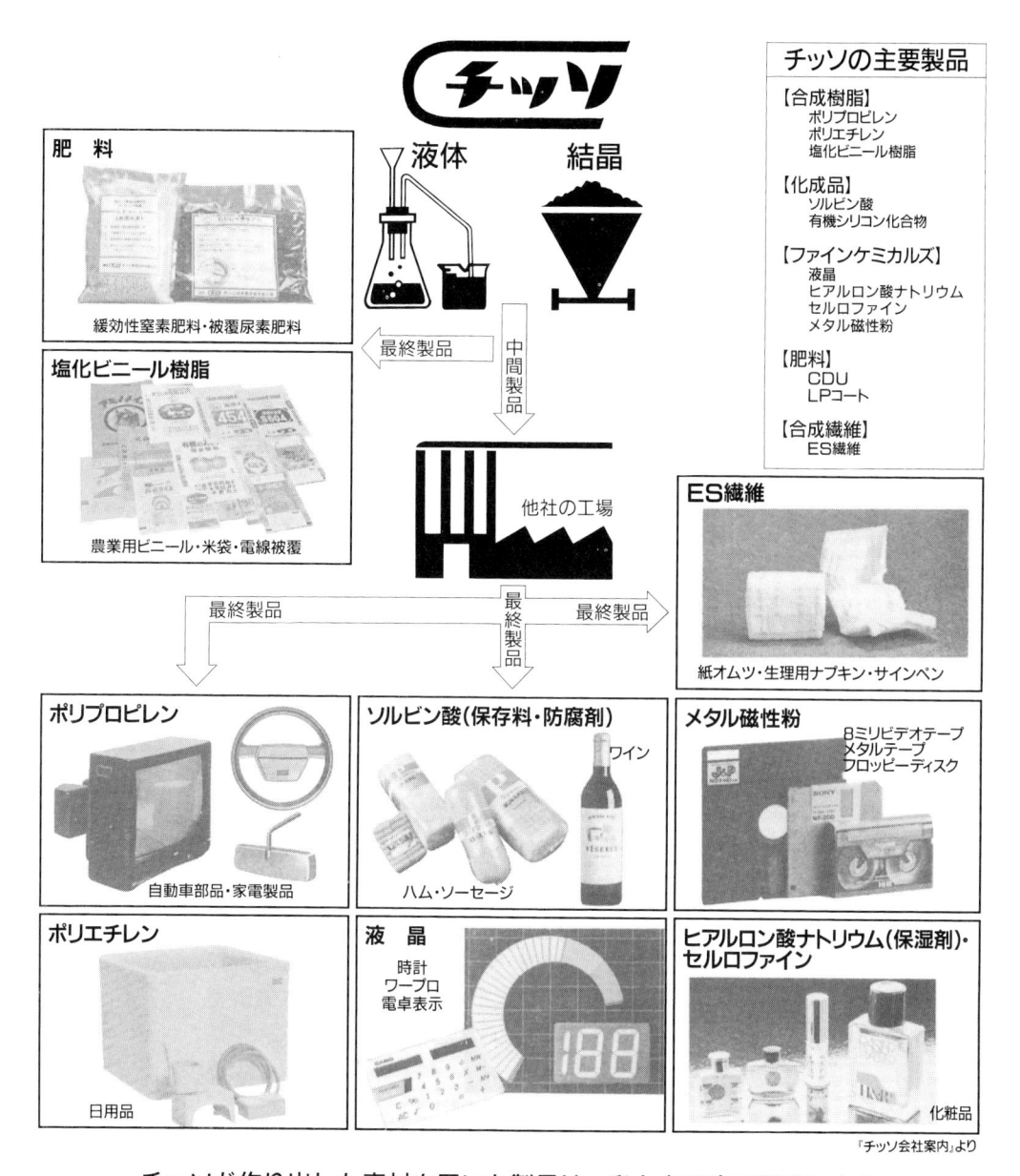

チッソの主要製品

【合成樹脂】
　ポリプロピレン
　ポリエチレン
　塩化ビニール樹脂

【化成品】
　ソルビン酸
　有機シリコン化合物

【ファインケミカルズ】
　液晶
　ヒアルロン酸ナトリウム
　セルロファイン
　メタル磁性粉

【肥料】
　CDU
　LPコート

【合成繊維】
　ES繊維

肥料 — 緩効性窒素肥料・被覆尿素肥料

塩化ビニール樹脂 — 農業用ビニール・米袋・電線被覆

ES繊維 — 紙オムツ・生理用ナプキン・サインペン

ポリプロピレン — 自動車部品・家電製品

ソルビン酸（保存料・防腐剤） — ハム・ソーセージ、ワイン

メタル磁性粉 — 8ミリビデオテープ、メタルテープ、フロッピーディスク

ポリエチレン — 日用品

液晶 — 時計、ワープロ、電卓表示

ヒアルロン酸ナトリウム（保湿剤）・セルロファイン — 化粧品

『チッソ会社案内』より

　チッソが作り出した素材を用いた製品は、私たちの身の回りにあふれている。チッソの技術は、私たちの生活を便利で快適なものにしてきた。チッソをはじめとする化学工業に支えられて経済成長を遂げた日本。しかし、発展に目を奪われた結果が水俣病である。

朝鮮チッソ興南工場

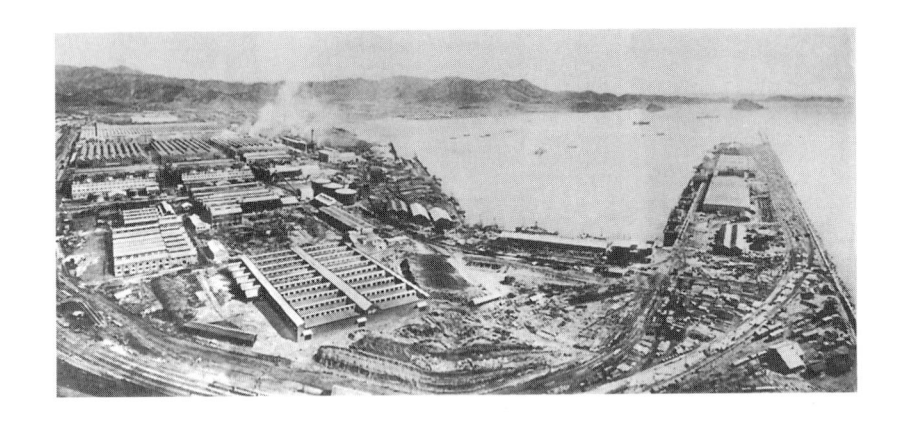

昭和初期、チッソは硫安の製造販売で得た利益を、朝鮮北部の興南工場建設に注いだ。日本軍による朝鮮占領の力に支えられ、人口約3000人はいたといわれる農漁村は巨大な工場群に一変した。豊かな資金で巨大なダムを次々につくり、電力を起こし、鉄道や病院、社員住宅などを建設。日本軍の力を借りて村民を強制立退きさせ、東洋一といわれる一大植民地（盛時人口20万人）を形成した。同時に、「工員は牛馬と思え」と現地の朝鮮人労働者に苛酷な労働を強いていた。

『日本窒素肥料事業大観』より

チッソ水俣工場

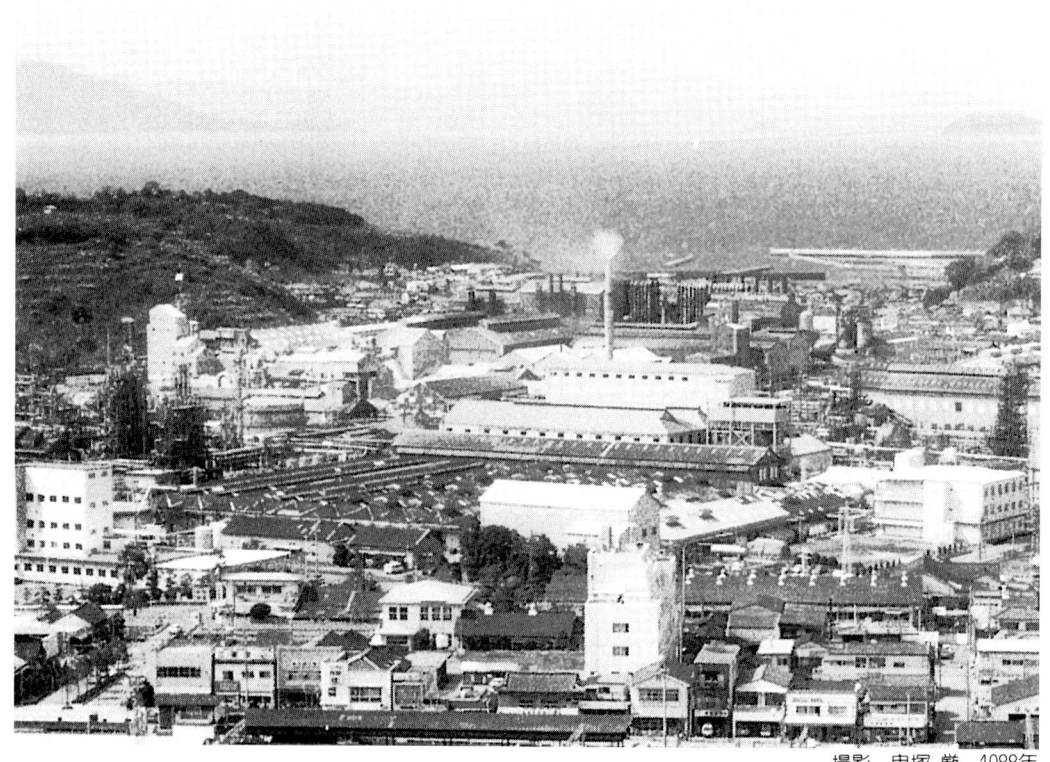

撮影　鬼塚巌　1988年

今も変わらず市の中心部に位置する、老朽化したチッソ水俣工場。盛時の面影をわずかにとどめるが、広大な用地のうち、工場として稼動しているのは、約5分の1に過ぎない。

水銀の流出とチッソの加害行為

水俣病は、チッソが水俣湾に無処理で流した廃水によって引き起こされた。廃水中のメチル水銀は、アセトアルデヒド製造のための触媒として使用されたもので、1932(昭和7)年より、実に36年間にわたって流された。1959(昭和34)年、原因がチッソの廃水であると究明されて以後も、なお9年間、水銀は流され続けた。現在も、水銀をはじめ大量の有害物質がヘドロとなって水俣湾周辺の海底に堆積し、不知火海全域に広がり続けている。

アセトアルデヒドを作るため水銀が使われた

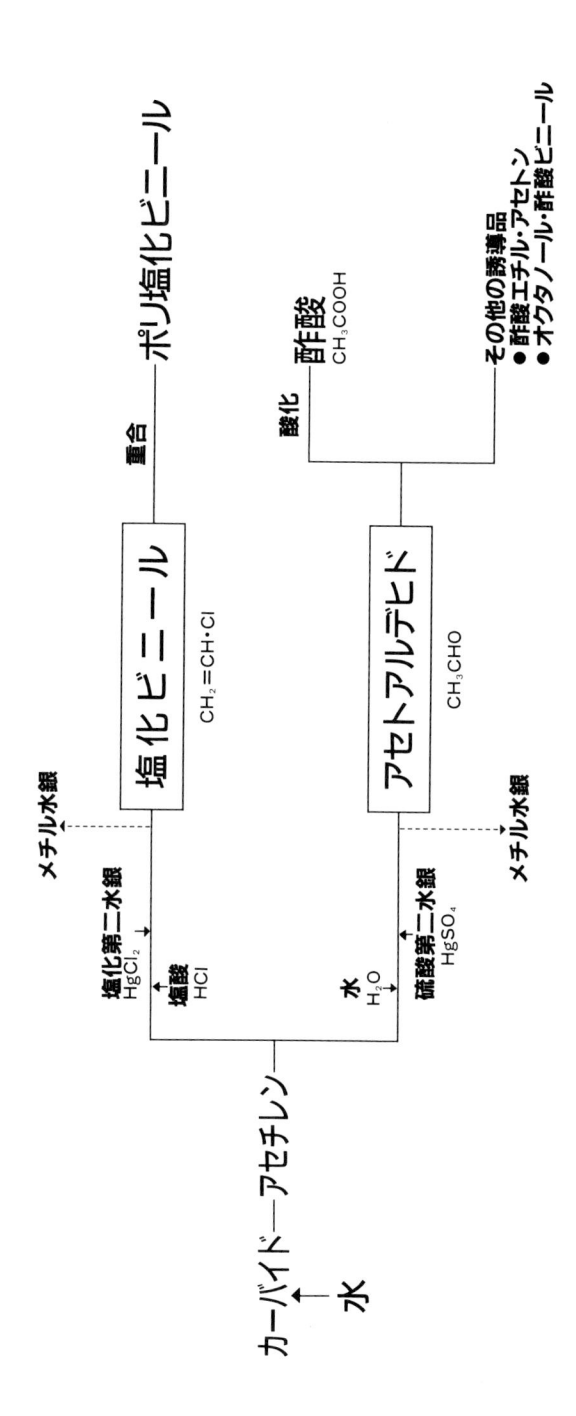

カーバイド → アセチレン
　　↑
　　水

塩化第二水銀 HgCl₂ ↓
塩酸 HCl →

塩化ビニール
CH₂=CH・Cl

重合 → ポリ塩化ビニール

メチル水銀

水 H₂O →
硫酸第二水銀 HgSO₄ ←

アセトアルデヒド
CH₃CHO

メチル水銀

酸化 → 酢酸 CH₃COOH

その他の誘導品
● 酢酸エチル・アセトン
● オクタノール・酢酸ビニール

チッソ水俣工場では、合成酢酸の原料、アセトアルデヒドをつくるための触媒として、硫酸水銀が用いられた。この過程で硫酸水銀が有機化してメチル水銀が副生される。重金属の水銀がもつ毒性の強さはよく知られているが、これがメチル化するとタンパク質と結びつきやすくなることから飛躍的に毒性が増す。メチル水銀は、結晶から直接揮発して、王子の腐ったようなにおいがする。

メチル水銀は工場から海へ

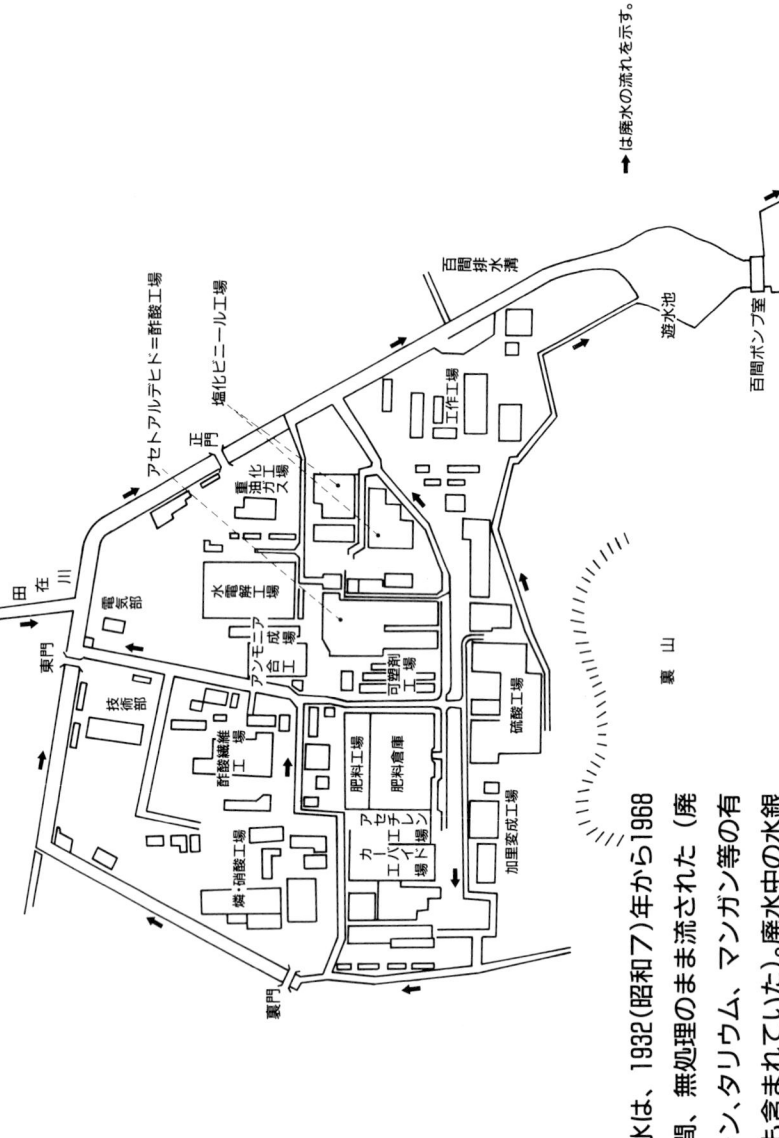

→は廃水の流れを示す。

[工場配置図：アセトアルデヒド＝酢酸工場、塩化ビニール工場、正門、重油タンク、電気部、水電解工場、アンモニア合成工場、司塑剤工場、硫酸工場、技術部、酢酸繊維工場、肥料工場、肥料倉庫、加里変成工場、カーバイド工場、エバポレーター工場、樟・硝酸工場、裏門、東門、田在川、百間排水溝、百間ポンプ室、遊水池、水俣港、工作工場、裏山]

メチル水銀を含んだ廃水は、1932(昭和7)年から1968(昭和43)年までの36年間、無処理のまま流された（廃水には、水銀以外にセレン、タリウム、マンガン等の有毒な重金属や化学物質も含まれていた）。廃水中の水銀は400～600トンにもおよび、海に拡がった水銀へドロを全部回収することは不可能といわれている。

魚のすみかが失われた

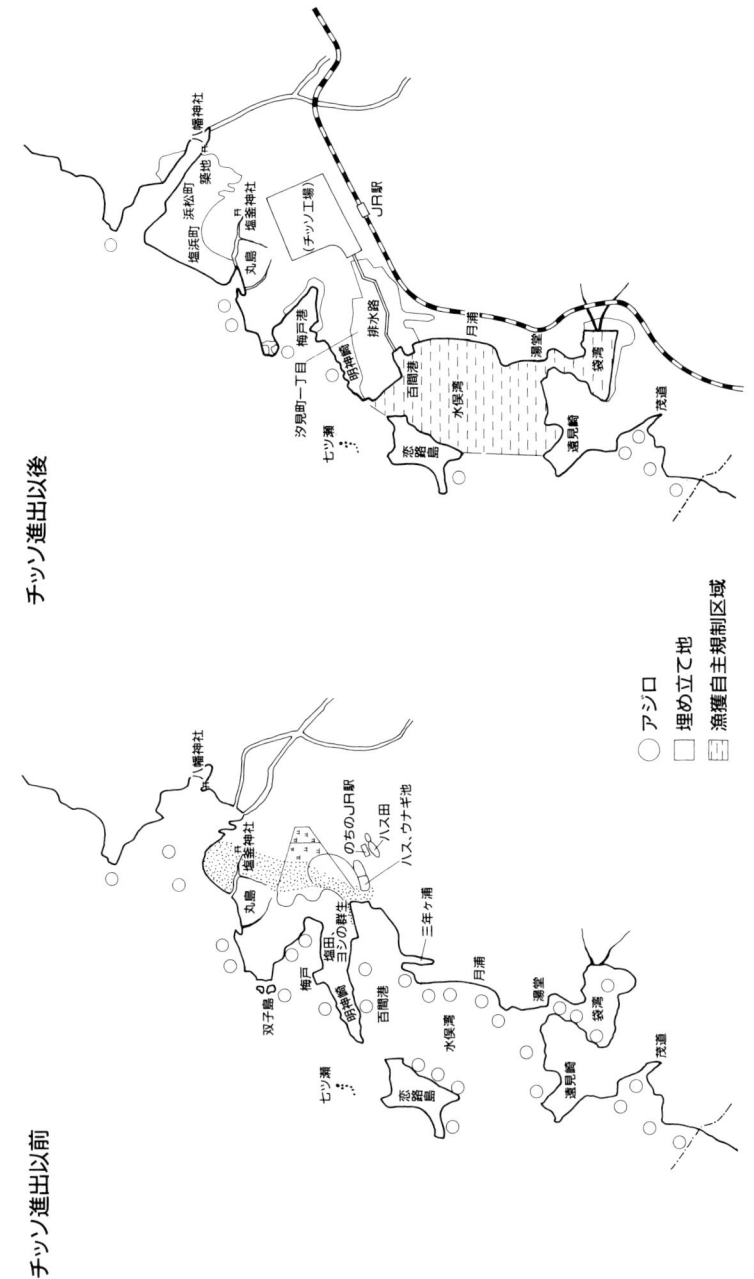

チッソ進出以前

チッソ進出以後

○ アジロ
□ 埋め立て地
☷ 漁獲自主規制区域

水俣湾やその回りの海岸には、「アジロ」と呼ばれ、魚たちの集まる場所がたくさんあった。廃水を流し続けて浅くなってしまった港を浚渫し、埋立てたり、廃水プールを作ったりしたために、アジロはほとんどなくなってしまった。豊かだった海はチッソによって死んでしまった。

チッソ城下町・水俣

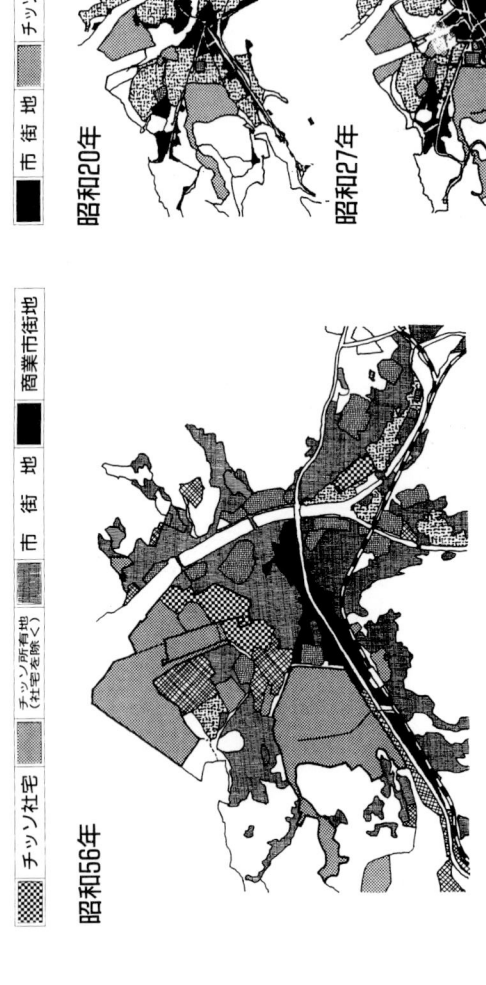

明治33年

明治44年

大正12年

昭和20年

昭和27年

昭和41年

昭和56年

チッソは、水俣に進出して以来、市の政治・経済の支配者としての色合を急速に強めていった。1950(昭和25)年には、水俣病の発端となった酢酸合成法を発明した橋本彦七・元水俣工場長が市長になっている。こうしたことは市街地の変化にも現れ、チッソ所有の土地は増加の一途をたどった。昭和60年代以降、チッソが八幡廃水プールを市に売却するなどしたため、現在は図に見られる1981(昭和56)年当時とは多少異なっている。

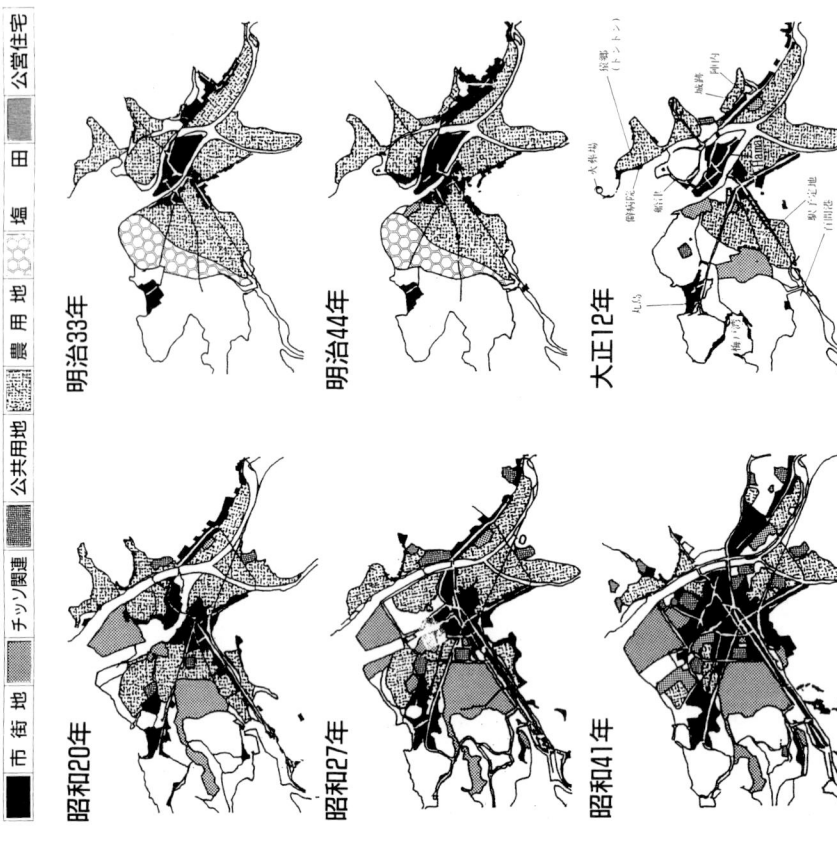

水銀は魚介類をへてひとへ

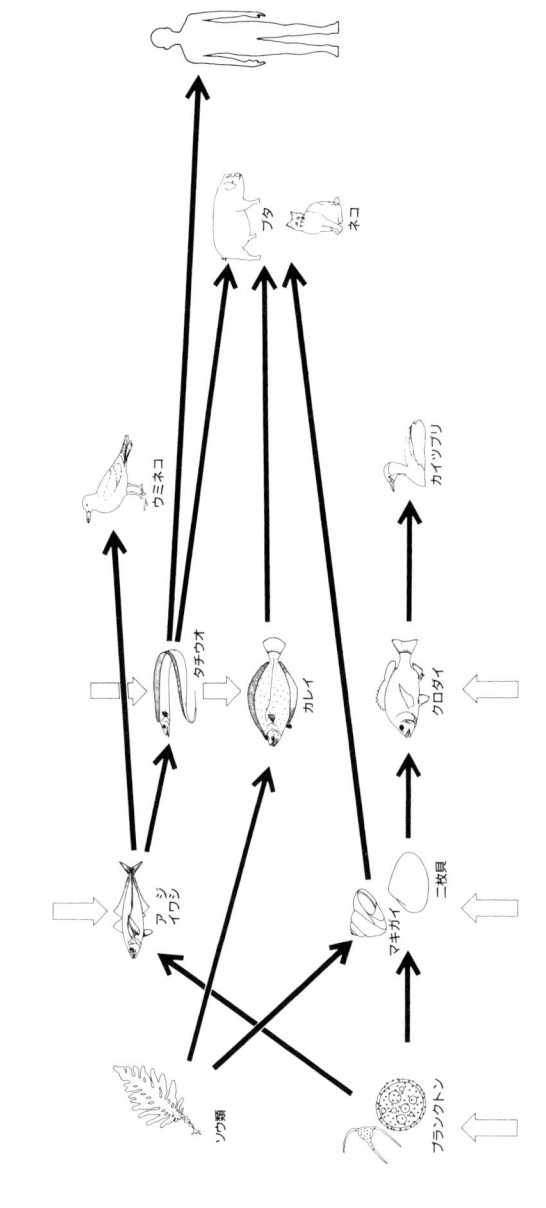

廃水とともに海に放出されたメチル水銀は海水で薄められるが、食物連鎖によってたちまち数万倍、数十万倍の濃さとなって生き物の体内にたまっていく。メチル水銀はプランクトンに吸収され、それを食う魚や貝が食べる。またメチル水銀は、魚のエラや体表からも直接吸収される。エサといっしょに泥を食べるような魚は、泥からもメチル水銀をとりこんでしまう。メチル水銀によって魚も水俣病になった。その魚をたべた鳥、猫、犬、豚など、そして最後には人間が発病した。人びとは「猫おどり病」「奇病」と呼んで恐れた。

健康被害

水俣病は、体内蓄積したメチル水銀によって主に脳の中枢神経系と末梢神経が冒される病気で、感覚障害、ふるえなど多彩な臨床症状を示す全身病である。水銀に汚染された魚を食べた人は数十万人におよぶといわれている。これら住民に対する潜在患者発掘のために、一斉検診の必要性が言われながら今日までまったくなされていない。

水銀が神経細胞を破壊する

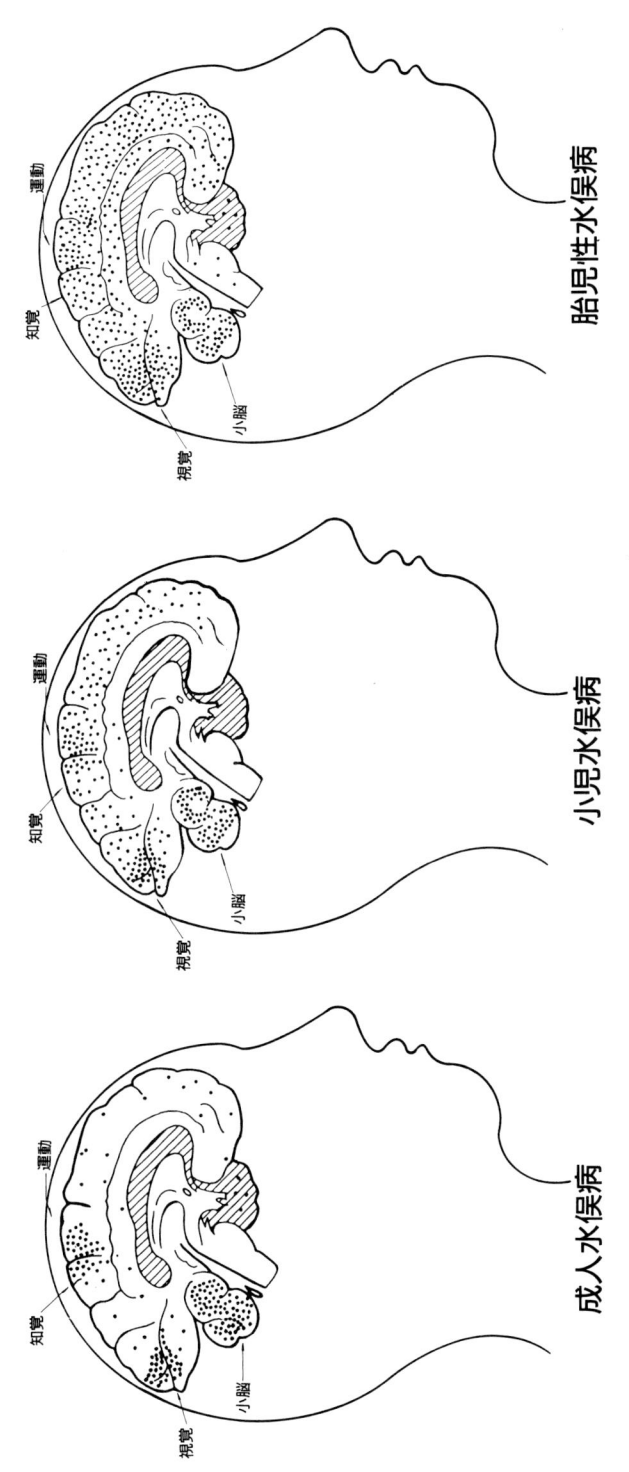

成人水俣病　　　　小児水俣病　　　　胎児性水俣病

運動／知覚／視覚／小脳

▨ はメチル水銀によって冒される部分

魚や貝をとおして体の中に入ったメチル水銀は、胃や腸から吸収され、脳や体全体に入る。脳に入ったメチル水銀は、脳を萎縮（小さく）させてしまう。神経細胞を冒し、体の平衡を保つ小脳や知覚（聴覚、視覚、触覚など）をつかさどる部分を特に破壊する。

母体を通して水銀は胎児へ

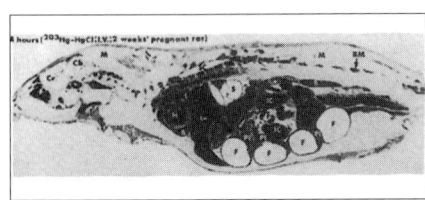

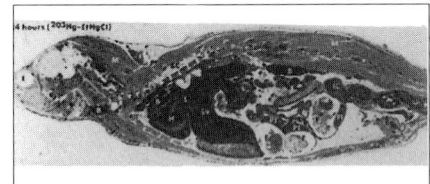

Fは胎児。黒い部分ほど水銀がたまっている。　2図

母親が食べた魚をとおして体に入ったメチル水銀は、母親の全身に回るだけでなく、へその緒でつながる胎児にも入ってゆく。上の1図は、妊娠2週目のネズミに、無機水銀（Hg-HCl・塩化水銀）を静脈注射して、24時間たったもの。2図は同じく妊娠2週目のネズミに、有機水銀（Hg-E＋HgCl・塩化エチル水銀）を注射して24時間たったもの。無機水銀はほとんど内蔵に集中しているが、有機水銀はほぼ全身に回り、脳へも侵入している。また有機水銀が、母親の胎盤をくぐり抜け、胎児にまで被害を与えている。

提供　白木博次

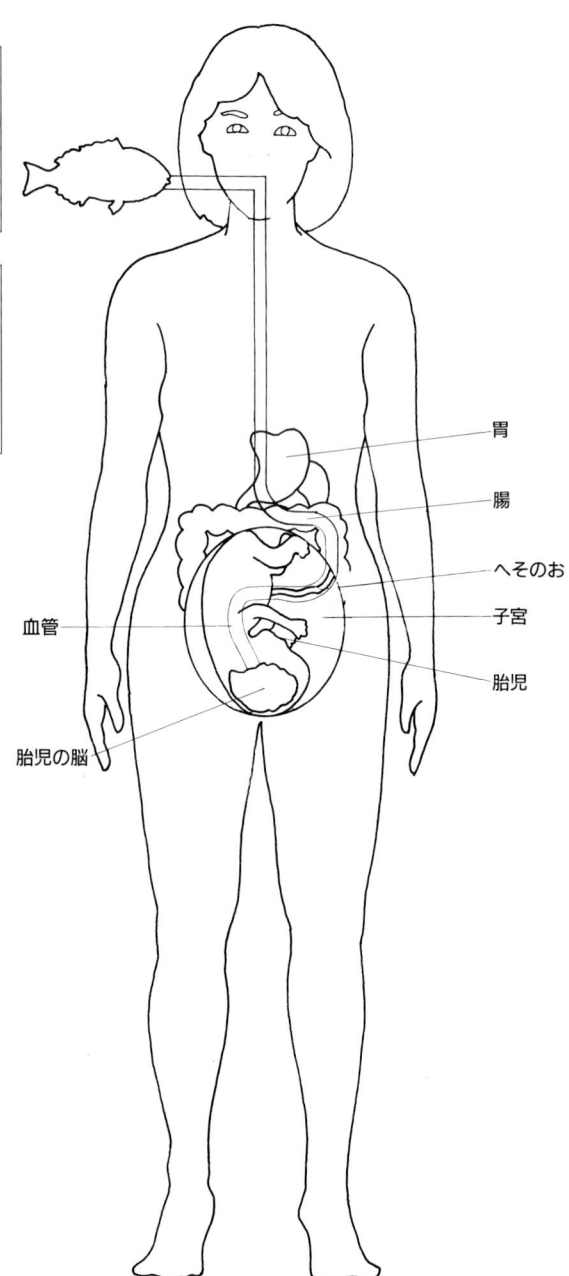

胃
腸
へそのお
子宮
胎児
血管
胎児の脳

全身に症状が

調査　六反田藤吉　1974年

患者が訴える自覚症状

症　　　状	男(%)	女(%)
物忘れ	85.9	83.6
力が入りにくい	80.4	75.2
歩きにくい	76.4	70.8
手，足のしびれ感	74.8	73.3
手，足先が不器用	72.4	67.0
手，足のふるえ	71.5	59.4
目が見えにくい	71.2	78.6
体がだるい	70.6	73.6
頭痛，頭重	66.9	70.4
首，肩，へきの痛み	64.7	74.2
腰　痛	63.8	63.2
ねむれない	62.6	69.8
耳が聞こえにくい	62.3	55.3
言葉のもつれ	61.0	51.3
ひきつけ　カラス曲り	60.7	64.2
めまい	56.1	62.3
耳鳴り	51.2	58.5
関節の痛み	47.9	50.6
体全体のしびれ感	36.8	36.2
体全体の痛み	33.7	28.6
全身のけいれん	29.1	31.4
よだれ	28.2	28.9
その他	5.5	6.6

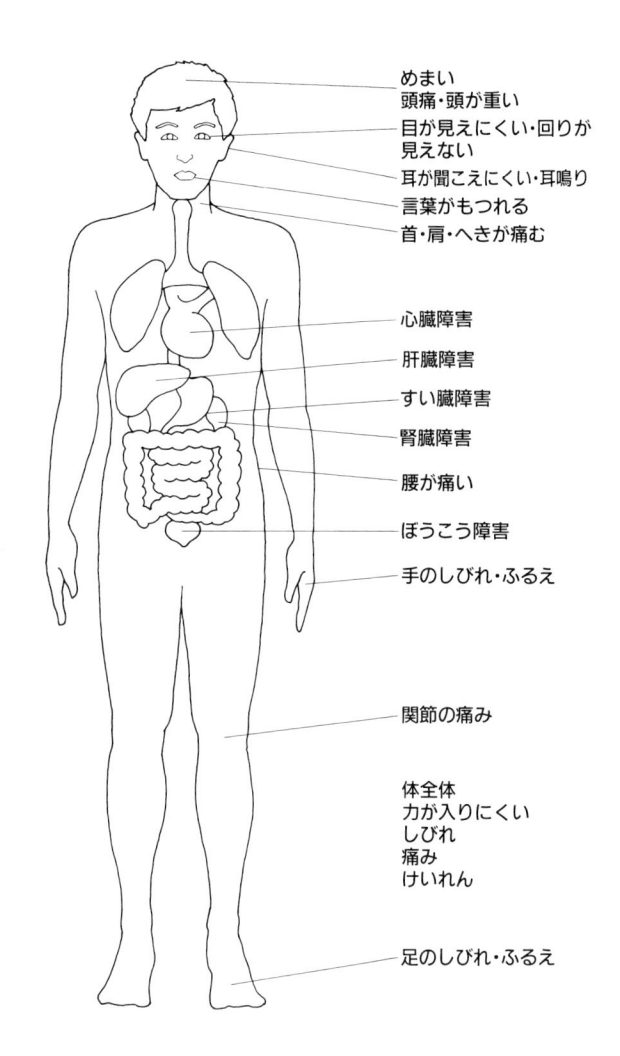

「水俣市並びにその周辺地域の医療需給に関する研究班」報告書より

- めまい
- 頭痛・頭が重い
- 目が見えにくい・回りが見えない
- 耳が聞こえにくい・耳鳴り
- 言葉がもつれる
- 首・肩・へきが痛む
- 心臓障害
- 肝臓障害
- すい臓障害
- 腎臓障害
- 腰が痛い
- ぼうこう障害
- 手のしびれ・ふるえ
- 関節の痛み
- 体全体　力が入りにくい　しびれ　痛み　けいれん
- 足のしびれ・ふるえ

水俣病は全身に影響をおよぼす。手足のしびれやふるえ、目の回りが見えなくなることなど、たくさんの症状がある。すい臓が悪くなって糖尿病になる人もいるなど、目に見えない被害は多い。こうした多くの症状を、水俣病の影響と認めない医者も多くいる。

書字障害

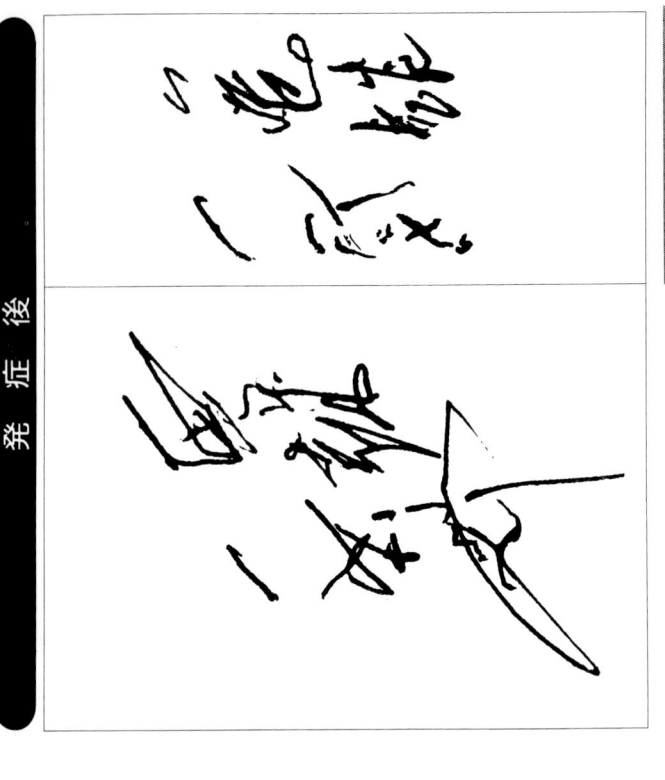

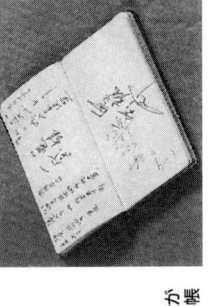

発症前

発症後

水俣病患者が使っていた手帳

水俣病患者が手帳に書き残した文字。字を書こうとすると手がふるえる。同じ人が書いたものとは思えないものになってしまう。病状が悪化するにつれ、字を書いたものとは思えないものになってしまう。魚の仲買をしていたこの患者は、1959年ごろ、医師から「水俣病ではないか」といわれて入院したが、漁業組合の人たちは「この村から患者が出たら魚が売れなくなる」といって、無理矢理、退院させてしまった。

苦痛は生活の中で拡大する

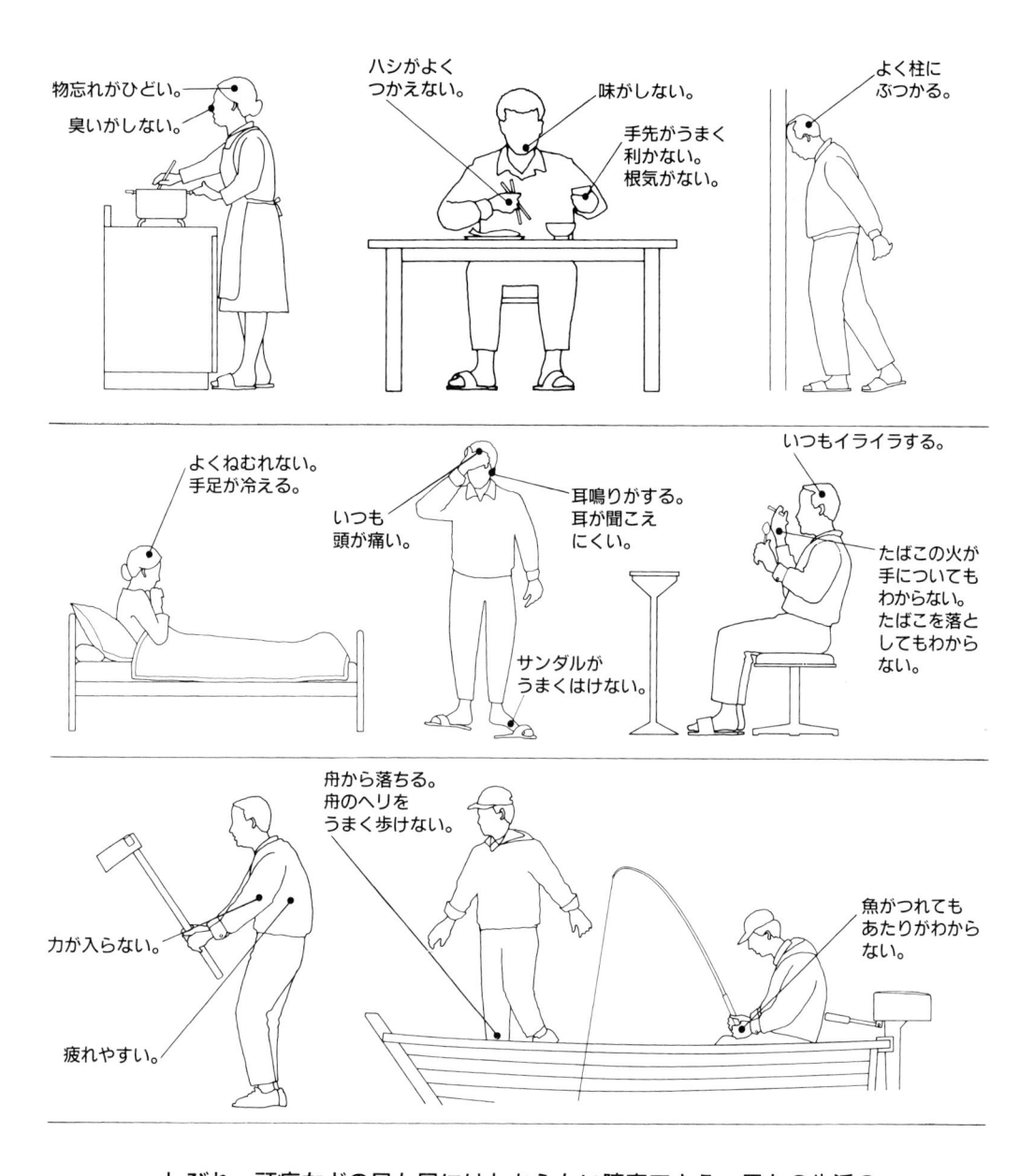

- 物忘れがひどい。
- 臭いがしない。
- ハシがよくつかえない。
- 味がしない。
- 手先がうまく利かない。根気がない。
- よく柱にぶつかる。
- よくねむれない。手足が冷える。
- いつも頭が痛い。
- 耳鳴りがする。耳が聞こえにくい。
- サンダルがうまくはけない。
- いつもイライラする。
- たばこの火が手についてもわからない。たばこを落としてもわからない。
- 力が入らない。
- 疲れやすい。
- 舟から落ちる。舟のヘリをうまく歩けない。
- 魚がつれてもあたりがわからない。

しびれ、頭痛などの見た目にはわからない障害でさえ、日々の生活の中では、ひとつひとつの動作に多大な影響を及ぼす。頭痛が続いて休んでいても「なまけもの」と非難される精神的な打撃も考えればその苦痛は、はかりしれない。

汚染は不知火海全域に広がった
―― 1960〜62年の毛髪水銀量調査 ――

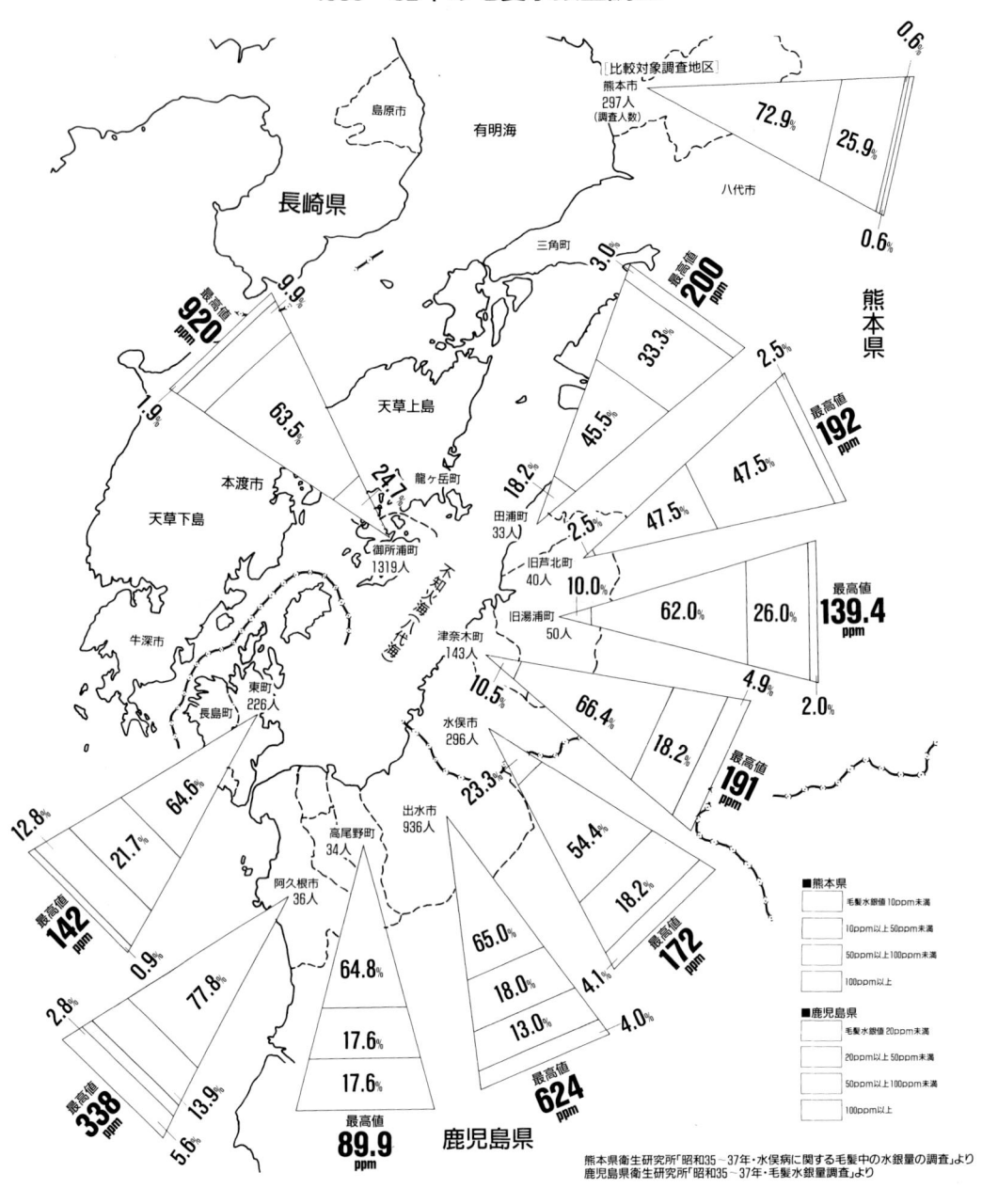

熊本県・鹿児島県は1960年ころ、不知火海南部沿岸の人びとの髪の毛を調査したが、この人びとの髪の毛には、多量の水銀が含まれていることがわかった。日本人は普通1〜5ppm程度と言われているが、中には920ppmもの値を示した人もいた。対象地区の熊本市に比べても、この地域の人々の水銀汚染のひどさがわかる。県は調査しただけで、その結果を住民に知らせることもせず、チッソは水銀廃水を流し続けた。

熊本県衛生研究所「昭和35〜37年・水俣病に関する毛髪中の水銀量の調査」より
鹿児島県衛生研究所「昭和35〜37年・毛髪水銀量調査」より

不知火海全域から水俣病申請患者が
水俣病認定申請者の増加

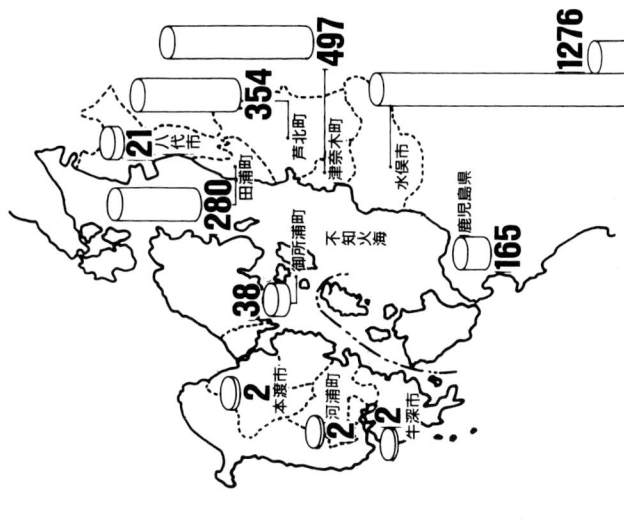

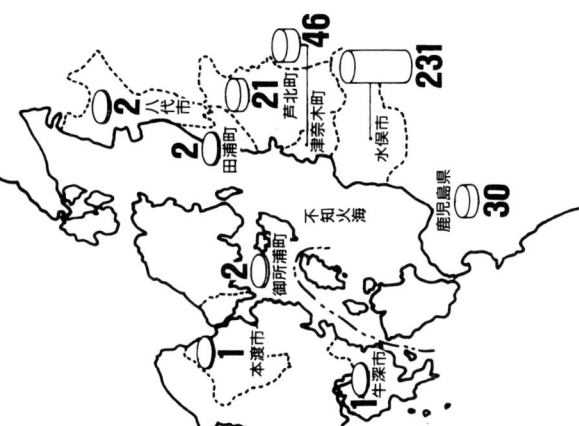

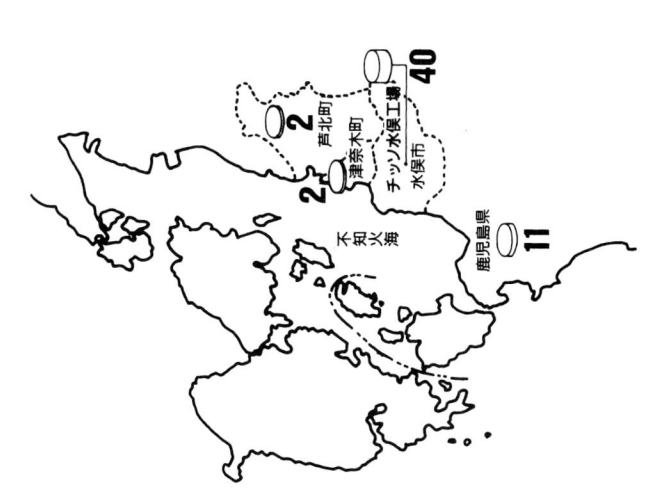

1961年

- 芦北町 2
- 津奈木町 2
- チッソ水俣工場/水俣市 40
- 鹿児島県 11

1971年

- 八代市 2
- 田浦町 2
- 芦北町 21
- 津奈木町 46
- 水俣市 231
- 御所浦町 2
- 本渡市 1
- 牛深市 1
- 鹿児島県 30

1973年

- 八代市 21
- 田浦町 280
- 芦北町 354
- 津奈木町 497
- 水俣市 1276
- 宮所浦町 38
- 本渡市 2
- 河浦町 2
- 牛深市 2
- 鹿児島県 165

数字は人数

チッソの水銀廃水は、南部不知火海の沿岸全域で人びとの健康を害した。人びとは水俣病に対する偏見や差別を恐れて、自らの病いを隠した。その上、行政もチッソに配慮して、水俣病を隠しつづけた。しかし、被害者自身の闘いによって、少しづつ水俣病に対する理解は広がり、水俣病患者としての認定を求める人は全地域におよんだ。

1979年

- 579
- 790
- 65
- 959
- 1500
- 7 本渡市
- 2 河浦町
- 5 牛深市
- 御所浦町
- 田浦町
- 八代市
- 芦北町
- 津奈木町
- 不知火海
- 水俣市
- 鹿児島県
- 2876
- 1578

1985年

- 1022
- 1164
- 89
- 1329
- 2199
- 13 本渡市
- 2 河浦町
- 6 牛深市
- 御所浦町
- 田浦町
- 八代市
- 芦北町
- 津奈木町
- 不知火海
- 水俣市
- 鹿児島県
- 3905
- 2928

1990年

- 1337
- 1350
- 105
- 1570
- 2609
- 15 本渡市
- 2 河浦町
- 11 牛深市
- 御所浦町
- 田浦町
- 八代市
- 芦北町
- 津奈木町
- 不知火海
- 水俣市
- 鹿児島県
- 4573
- 3702

20万人以上の被害者が裾野に拡がっている

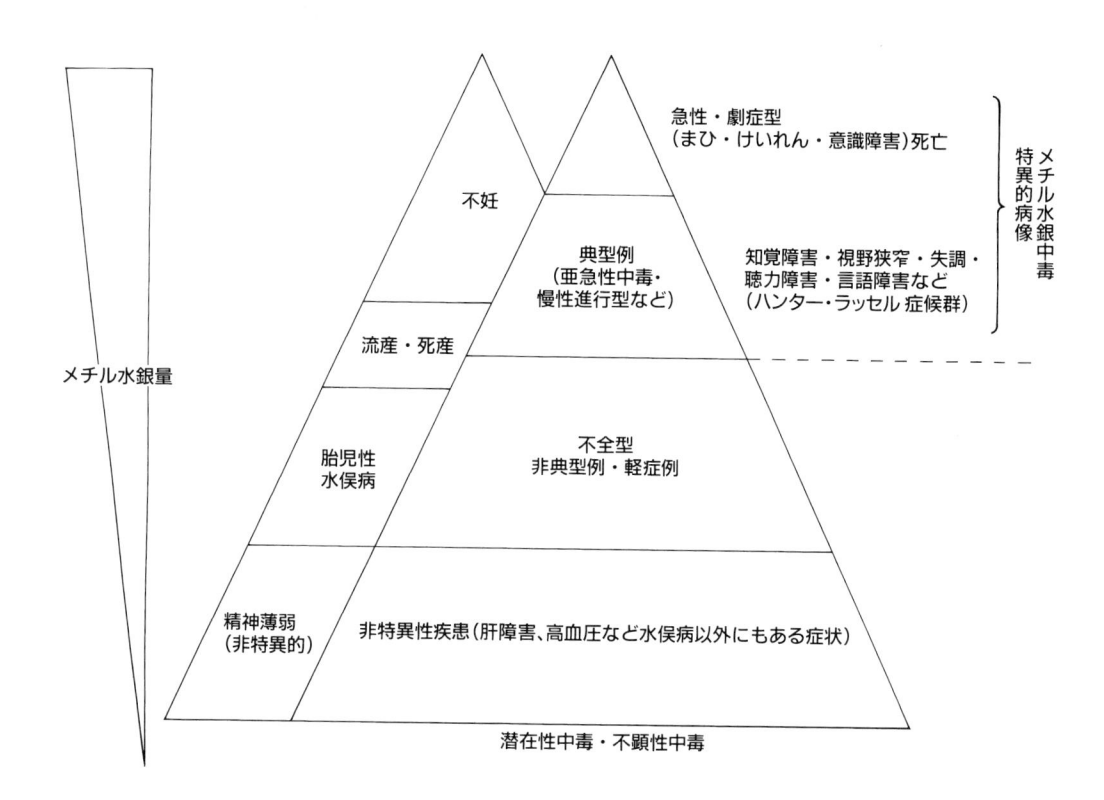

メチル水銀量

急性・劇症型
(まひ・けいれん・意識障害)死亡

知覚障害・視野狭窄・失調・
聴力障害・言語障害など
(ハンター・ラッセル症候群)

}特異的病像 メチル水銀中毒

不妊

典型例
(亜急性中毒・
慢性進行型など)

流産・死産

胎児性
水俣病

不全型
非典型例・軽症例

精神薄弱
(非特異的)

非特異性疾患(肝障害、高血圧など水俣病以外にもある症状)

潜在性中毒・不顕性中毒

「ハンター・ラッセル症候群」と呼ばれる、イギリスの農薬工場労働者の有機水銀中毒例がある。その主な症状は、運動失調(字がうまく書けない、歩けない等)、感覚障害(手足のしびれ)、聴力障害(耳が聞こえない)、構音障害(うまくしゃべれない)、求心性視野狭窄(回りが見えない)、振顫(ふるえ)である。この症例を手がかりとして、水俣病の原因が有機水銀中毒と確認された。しかしこのことから、「この症状のものだけが水俣病」と間違った理解をする医学者も多くいた。実際には直接浴びた場合と環境の媒介があるのとではその症状も異なる。水俣病の症状は多様であり、「不全型」「非典型例」「軽症例」などがいわゆる「典型例」よりも多い。 さらに、他地域と比較すると、沿岸住民の体力や健康は大きなかたよりを見せ、水俣病の裾野の広さを物語っている。

被害は病苦を越えて

調査　富樫貞夫・丸山定巳（熊本大学）1981年

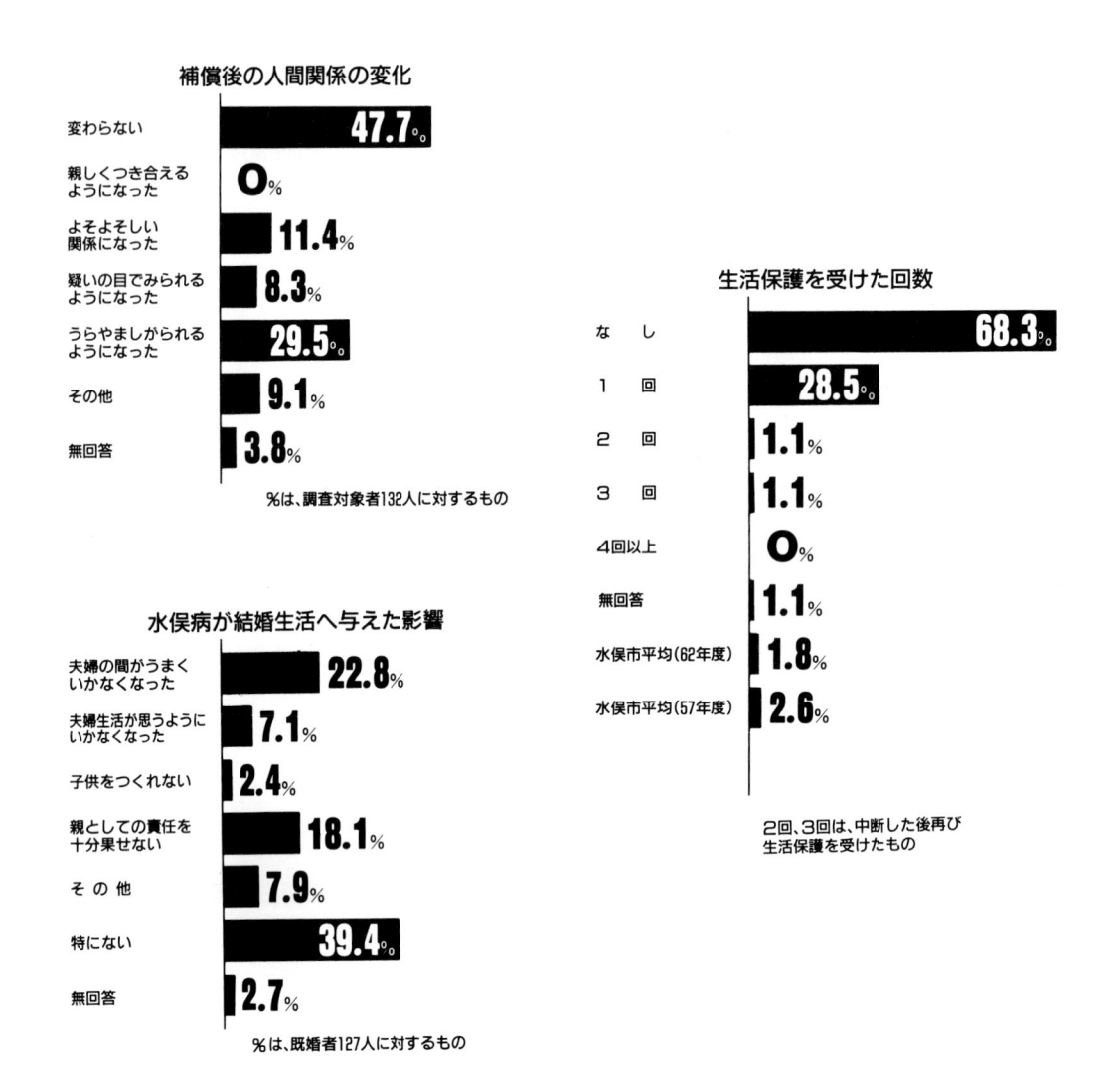

補償後の人間関係の変化

- 変わらない　47.7%
- 親しくつき合えるようになった　0%
- よそよそしい関係になった　11.4%
- 疑いの目でみられるようになった　8.3%
- うらやましがられるようになった　29.5%
- その他　9.1%
- 無回答　3.8%

%は、調査対象者132人に対するもの

生活保護を受けた回数

- な　し　68.3%
- 1　回　28.5%
- 2　回　1.1%
- 3　回　1.1%
- 4回以上　0%
- 無回答　1.1%
- 水俣市平均（62年度）　1.8%
- 水俣市平均（57年度）　2.6%

2回、3回は、中断した後再び生活保護を受けたもの

水俣病が結婚生活へ与えた影響

- 夫婦の間がうまくいかなくなった　22.8%
- 夫婦生活が思うようにいかなくなった　7.1%
- 子供をつくれない　2.4%
- 親としての責任を十分果せない　18.1%
- その他　7.9%
- 特にない　39.4%
- 無回答　2.7%

%は、既婚者127人に対するもの

被害者にとっては、健康を害されたことによる苦痛とともに、自分が思うようには生きられなくなったという苦痛が大きい。働き盛りに仕事ができなくなったり、近所や親戚縁者に疎まれたり、結婚や就職における差別があったり。水俣が「チッソ城下町」であるがゆえにこれらの被害は今なお根深く残る。

患者はどのような治療をしているのか

調査　富樫貞夫・丸山定巳（熊本大学）　1981年

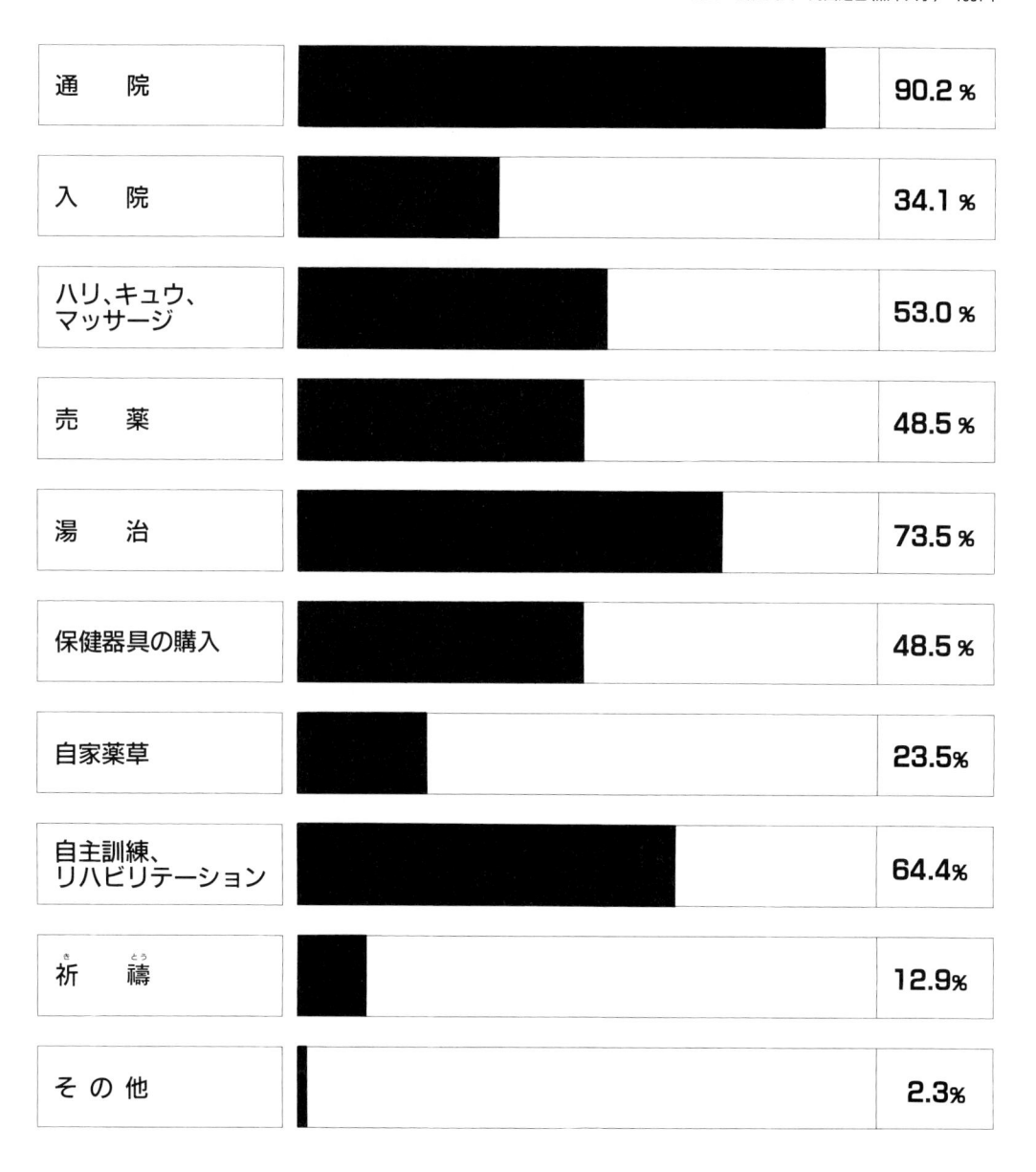

治療	割合
通院	90.2%
入院	34.1%
ハリ、キュウ、マッサージ	53.0%
売薬	48.5%
湯治	73.5%
保健器具の購入	48.5%
自家薬草	23.5%
自主訓練、リハビリテーション	64.4%
祈禱(きとう)	12.9%
その他	2.3%

　患者は、高令化による症状の悪化や不安にさらされている。「水俣病は治らない」といわれている。しかし、発病以来数十年を経過した現在でも、日々の痛苦を少しでも和らげようと病院に通ったり、治療器具をそろえるなど、さまざまな回復への努力を続けている。

多様な被害

水俣病患者の苦しみは、健康被害にとどまらない。チッソの廃水によって、漁民は仕事場である海を奪われ、生きがいと収入の道を断たれた。さらに「奇病」「伝染病」などと近隣の人びとからいわれのない差別を受け、大人ばかりでなく、子供は教育の、青年は就職や結婚の機会まで奪われた。健康被害に加えたこのような経済的打撃や差別によって、家庭さえ崩壊したところも珍しくない。水俣病は、患者の全生活を破壊したのである。

政治家たちの患者非難

> 認定申請者の中には補償金目当てのニセ患者がたくさんいる。もはや金の亡者だ。
>
> 熊本県議会議員（水俣市選出）　斉所一郎　一九七五（昭和50）年

> 認定審査会は、こうしたニセモノとホンモノを見分けるのに苦労している。運転免許の際は視野狭窄じゃないのに、検診の時は視野狭窄で見えないと答えている。
>
> 熊本県議会議員（公害対策特別委員会委員長・医師）　杉村国夫　一九七五（昭和50）年

> いま（明水園で）会った患者さんたちもかなりIQが低いわけですね。この手紙は非常にしっかりした文章というか、あるタイプの文章に見えますけど、これはやっぱり彼女たちが書いたんですかね。
>
> 環境庁長官　石原慎太郎　一九七七（昭和52）年

> 熊本県では、申請すれば水俣病患者になって、カネがもらえるから、そのうちに県民全部が水俣病患者になる。私も熊本県に住んで水俣病患者になりたい。
>
> 参議院議員（自民党政調会環境部会長）　森下　泰　一九七九（昭和54）年

被害者の救済に努力すべき政治家からも、水俣病患者や申請者に対して、悪口や非難が繰り返されている。政治的意図をもってなされるこうした人びとの発言は、世論に影響を与え、被害者への偏見や差別をより強くしている。

こんな言葉が投げつけられた

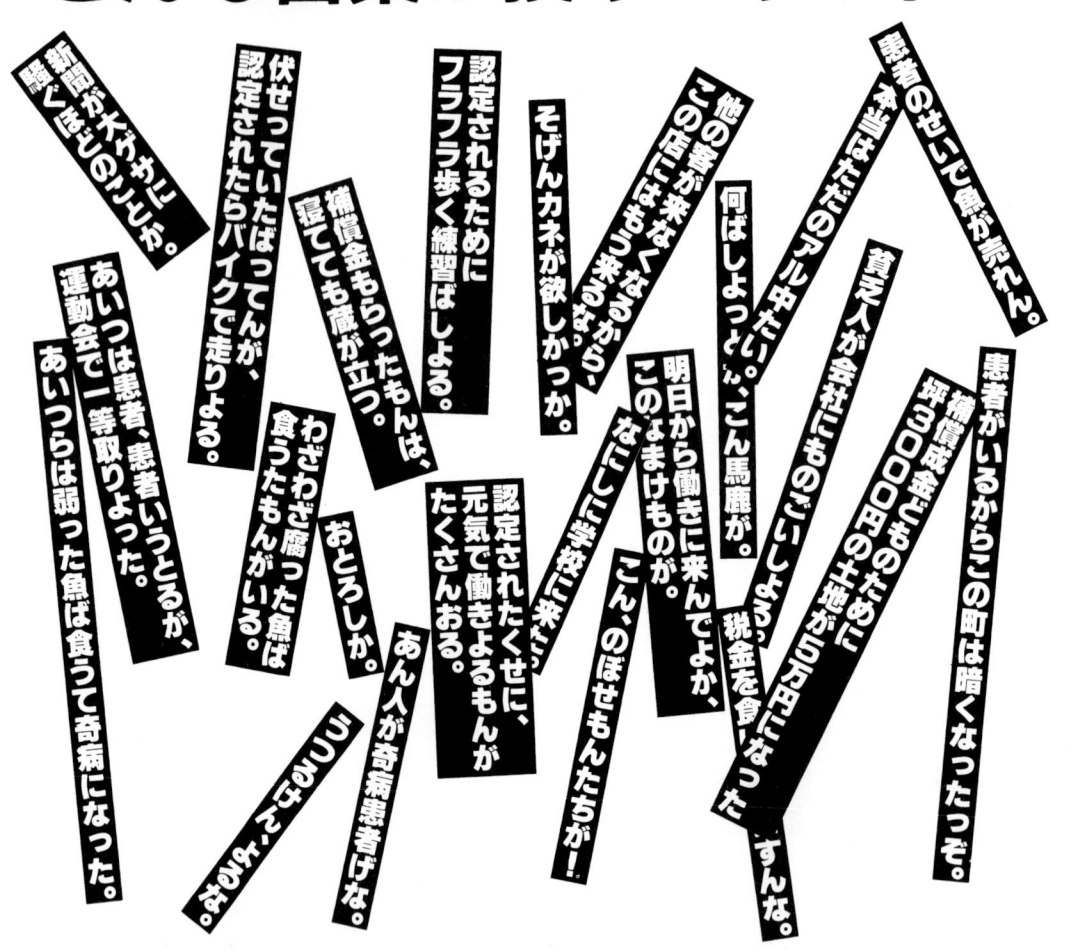

- 新聞が大げさに騒ぐほどのことか。
- 伏せっていたばってん、認定されたらバイクで走りよる。
- 認定されるためにフラフラ歩く練習ばしよる。
- 補償金もらったもんな、寝ても蔵が立つ。
- そげんカネが欲しかっか。
- 他の客が来なくなるから、この店にはもう来るな。
- 患者のせいで魚が売れん。
- 神様当はただのアル中たい。
- 何ばしよっと、こん馬鹿が。
- 貧乏人が会社にものごいしよって。
- 明日から働きに来んでよか、このよまけものが。
- なにしに学校に来た、こん、のぼせもんたちが！
- 税金を食うとるな。
- 患者がいるからこの町は暗くなったっぞ。
- 補償成金どものために坪3000円の土地が5万円になったぞ。
- あいつは患者、患者いうとるが、運動会で一等取りよった。
- あいつらは弱った魚は食うて奇病になった。
- わざわざ腐った魚は食うたもんがいる。
- おとろしか。
- 認定されたくせに、元気で働きよるもんがたくさんおる。
- あん人が奇病患者げな。
- うつるさな。

水俣病が発見された頃、患者は「奇病」「伝染病」とののしられ、兄弟や親類さえ家に寄りつかないという目にあった。

長い闘いの末に、水俣病患者はチッソから補償金を勝ちとってきたが補償金は一方で、悪質な中傷やねたみを招く、新たな苦痛の一因になった。認定申請が相次ぐ頃になると、「ニセ患者」などと非難を浴びせられるようになった。手足の変形や寝たきり状態だけを水俣病と捉える「無知」や、補償金欲しさに患者はウソをつくという「偏見」が、残酷な視線を生み出す。

不知火海の魚を食べた人々がすべて汚染されている。――これが現実であり、水俣病はチッソが作り出した「犯罪」であるという事実を知らせることからしか、このような患者への暴言は消えない。

闘い──被害者の30年
3

原因究明期

水俣病は当初、原因不明の「奇病」として扱われた。その存在が細川医師によって報告されたのち、熊本大学により原因は工場廃水に汚染された魚の摂食と判明した。魚が売れなくなり、困窮を極めた漁民は廃水停止を求めてチッソに押しかけたが、低額の漁業補償で片づけられた。一方、熊本大学により、原因物質が水銀と判明したが、チッソは廃水が原因とは認めず、患者の補償も見舞金というかたちで処理された。原因者はあいまいのまま患者の発生も終ったとされ、その後も水銀の排出は続いてゆく。

まず猫が狂い死にをした
─1954(昭和29)年─

猫てんかんで全滅
ねずみの激増に悲鳴

水俣市
茂道部落

三十一日水俣市茂道漁業石本貫重さん(竺)は市衛生課を訪れ、ねずみが急増して漁村を荒し回り、手がつけられないと駆除方を申し込んだ。

同部落は直二十戸の漁村だが、不思議なことに六月初めごろから急に猫が狂い死し始め(部落ではねこテンカンといっている)百余匹いた猫がほとんど全滅してしまい、反対にねずみが急増、大威張りで部落中を荒し回り、被害はますます増大する一方、あわてた人々は各方面から猫を貰ってきたが、これまた気が狂ったようにキリキリ舞して死んでしまうというので逐に市に泣きついてきたものと判った。

なお同地区は水田はなく農業の関係なども見られず、不思議がるやら気味悪るがるやら衛生課でもねずみ退治にのり出すことになった。

1954(昭和29)年8月1日 熊本日日新聞

この前年頃から、魚や鳥や猫の変死が観察されている。茂道部落では、部落中の猫が姿を消した。不知火海の生き物の異変についての初の報道。

水俣病が発見された
―1956（昭和31）年―

水俣市字月浦附近に発生せる小児奇病について

昭和三十一年五月四日
水俣発第八四一号
熊本県水俣保健所長
（熊本県）衛生部長殿

水俣市字月浦附近に発生せる小児奇病について

五月一日水俣日窒附属病院小児科医師よりの通知により月浦附近に発生せる小児奇病について調査す。

一、患者田□静□六歳

本年三月末日頃感冒様症状にて軽度の発熱あり、四月十四日前後より手及び足の強直性麻痺症状現はれ、毎夜不眠となり泣き続け、殆ど食餌をとらずヤクルト一日一本位を摂取し、漸次すい弱す。二十三日窒附属病院小児科に入院す。症状は手及び足の強直性また言語発音不明瞭であり、入院以来殆ど食餌をとらざるに依り鼻腔より栄養を摂取しめたり。入院以来殆ど平熱、無欲状態。病院の検査成績、膝蓋反射亢進、バビンスキー反応（＋）、ケルニッヒー反応（－）、頸部硬直なし、脊髄液検査水様透明、パンデー僅々なり細胞数3。本患者が一番重症である。

二、田□実□三歳

姉静子と殆ど同様の症状あるも軽度にして入院せず。

三、田□静□のごく附近の子供

患者松□ふ□え七歳の症状（五月二日実母の話）

発病の経過

本年四月五日頃麻疹様病状発疹ありたり、最も熱の高い時三十七度三分位。

四月十一日水俣市袋町市川医院にて受診し所小児麻痺と言はれる。
四月十六日水俣市立病院小児科にて栄養失調と診断さる。
四月十七日水俣市浮地医院において脳性ひと言はれる。
四月三十日より日窒附属病院小児科に外来受診中。主なる症状は足及び手の強直性まひ症状で進行々々にて見らる。

なお患者田□静□は現在視力もおとろへ眼前二十cm位の手動は見にくい。眼前五十cm位の手動はかへって見易い。水俣市谷川医師（眼科）視神経萎縮症になるかもしれないと言ふ。

日窒附属病院入院患者田□静□の実母よりの直接聴取せる患者自宅附近の同類及び類似患者の情報について。

一、本年一月頃より患者宅の猫及び近所の猫が次き次きにけいれんを起して死亡す。発病より十日位して火の中に入ったり水の中に入ったり海中にとび込んで死亡したりする。計五、六匹。

一、田□静□自宅の近所

米森さんの子供三人中六歳の男子は昨年七月から小児麻痺と言はれ現在両手屈曲のま、強直状態である。

一、田□静□隣の江□下さんの女子七歳は、一、二日前より手足が悪く静□と同様の症状にて発病している。

一、近所の人川□千□吉五十五歳位は、一昨年より足がきかなくなり次に手がきかなくなり口もきかなくなり発狂し現在熊本市の精神病院に入院して居る。

一、同じ近所の山□数□小学三年生、昨年七月頃より水俣市尾田医院にて小児麻痺と言はれ死亡し之を看病した叔父さんも間もなく発病して同様の症状にて死亡した。

一、同じ近所と同一の井戸水を使用しその井戸水に何か中毒性の有害物があるのではないかと、七日井戸水を県衛生研究所に検査依頼した。

患者家族は附近十軒位と同一の井戸水を使用しその井戸水に何か中毒性の有害物があるのではないかと、七日井戸水を県衛生研究所に検査依頼した。

以上

故・細川一チッソ附属病院長
水俣病患者の発見者。チッソ社内での実験で、酢酸工場廃水をエサにまぜ、1959（昭和34）年実験ネコ400号を発病させることに成功。
撮影　ユージン・スミス

チッソ附属病院を訪れていた患者を、細川一院長らが「今まで見たこともない患者」として保健所に連絡した。公式に水俣病患者が発見された1956（昭和31）年5月1日である。まもなく、水俣保健所、水俣市立病院、地元医師などにより海辺の部落の調査が始まった。小さな部落から何人もの患者が出たので、「伝染病患者」として疑われ、隔離されてしまった。その後、熊本大学などの研究により「チッソの廃水中に含まれる水銀が原因」とされたが、「伝染病」「汚いもの」といったイメージは今日まで持ち続けられ、患者にとっていわれのない被害を幾重にも重ねてしまっている。

汚染魚は放置された
―1957（昭和32）年―

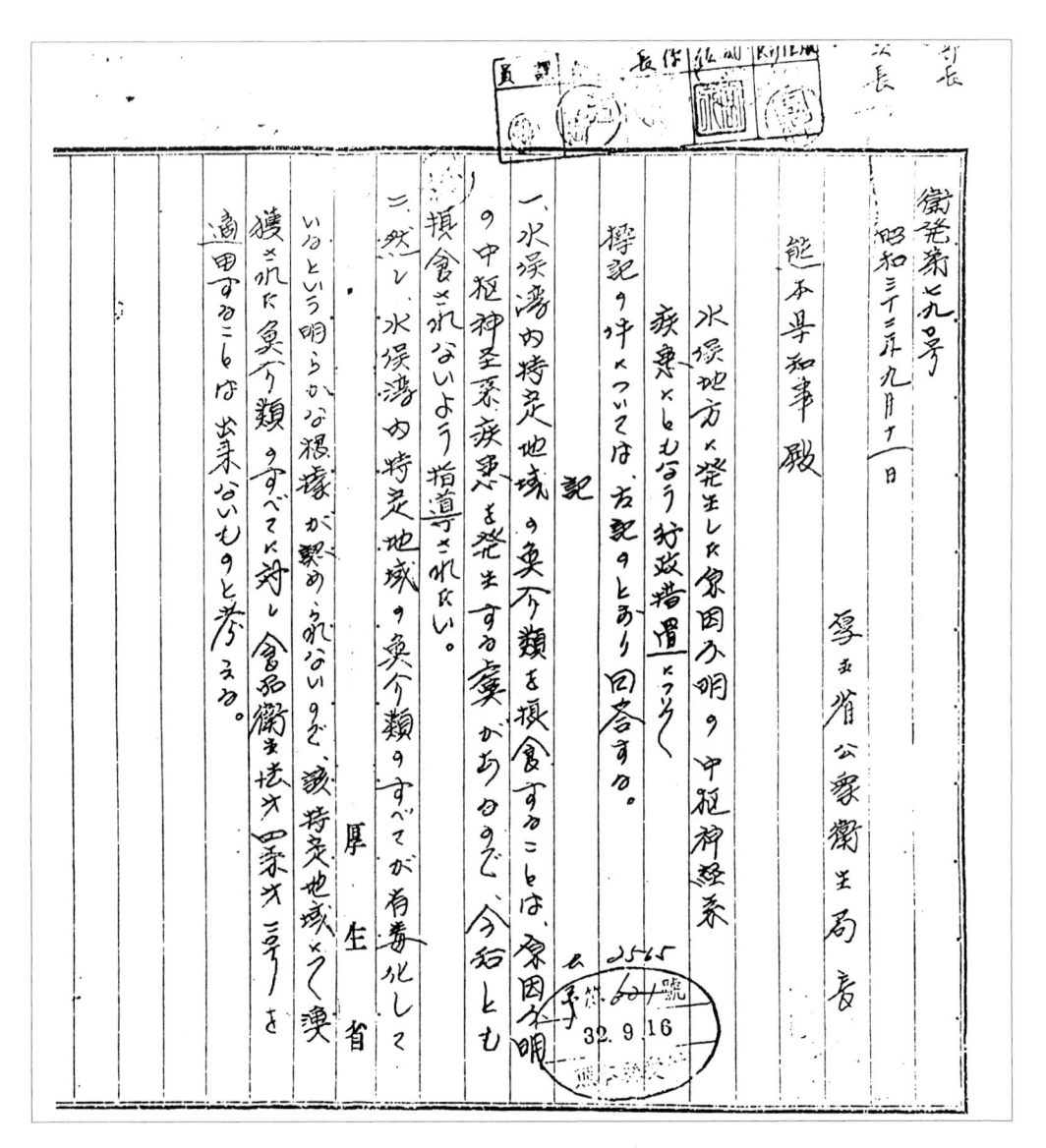

水俣湾の魚が原因で病気になることが、次第に明らかになってきたが、厚生省は法律で「魚を捕ってはいけない」と決めることをしなかった。この時以来、今日まで水俣湾内の魚は、法律で捕ることを禁止されたことは一度もない。漁民の人達が自分達で「捕らないようにしよう」と決めただけだった。それもいつの間にか「だいじょうぶだ」と言われて、1973（昭和48）年に第三水俣病事件が起きるまで再び水俣湾内の魚は捕られ、人びとに食べられていた。

漁民は立ち上った
──1959（昭和34）年──

1959（昭和34）年10月18日　熊本日日新聞

漁民デモで投石騒ぎ
保安員六人がケガ
工場長に決議文渡す

1959（昭和35）年11月3日　熊本日日新聞

漁民水俣で暴力ふるう
工場内に再度乱入
団交拒否に怒り爆発
警官と衝突　百余人が負傷

1959（昭和34）年　9月30日　湯浦漁協決議文

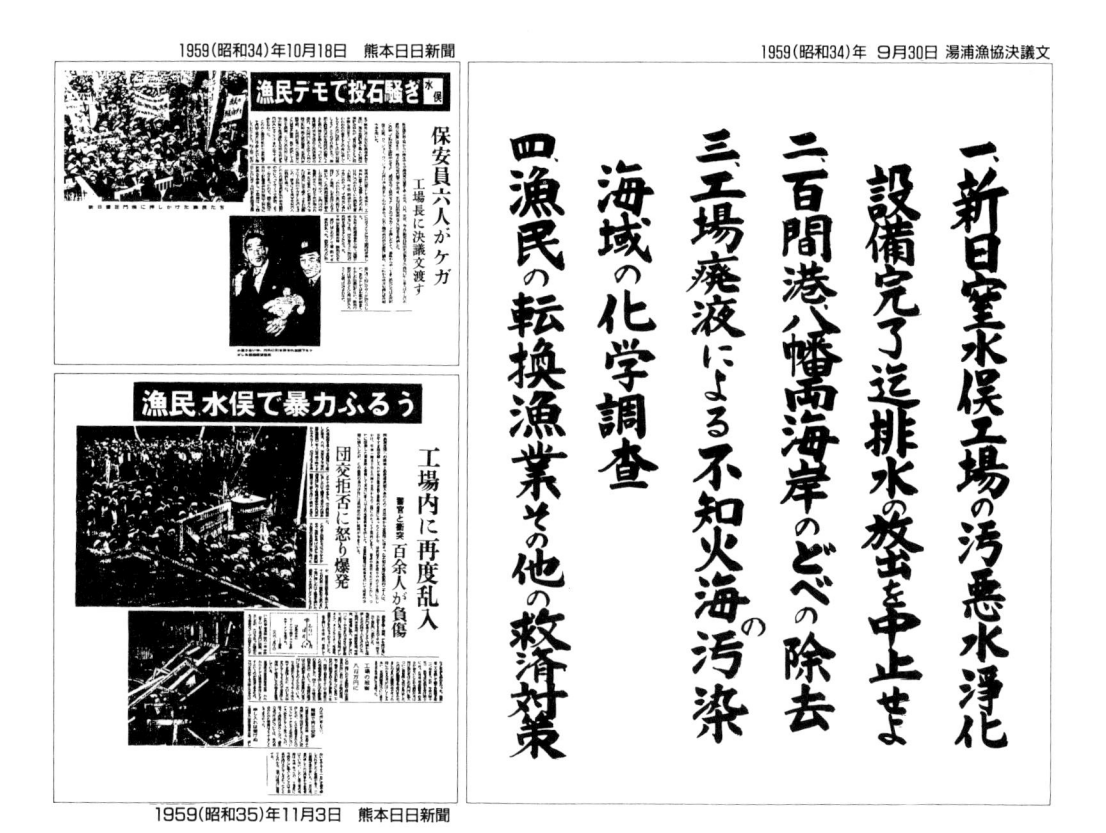

一、新日窒水俣工場の汚悪水浄化設備完了迄排水の一切を中止せよ
二、百間港、八幡両海岸のどべの除去
三、工場廃液による不知火海汚染海域の化学調査
四、漁民の転換漁業その他の救済対策

　不知火海における漁業被害は、チッソの創業とともに始まったといえる。1925（大正14）年には漁民がチッソに対して補償要求を行っている。チッソの廃水によって「魚が捕れない、捕っても売れない」という被害を受けたのは、不知火海全部の漁民だった。「汚れた水を流すな」と会社に押しかけ、補償を要求したが、逆に漁民が警察に逮捕されてしまった。チッソは廃水が原因で水俣病が発生（ネコ400号実験）することを隠し、「原因が工場廃水と決定しても追加補償しない」とし１億円の補償で済ませてしまった。不知火海漁民にとって、廃水停止が根本的な要求であった。

患者たちはやっと立ち上った
―1959（昭和34）年―

決議文

昭和二十八年頃より発生したる水俣病は、貴工場の排水に依って発病し死亡したる事は社会的事実であります。依って被害者七十八名の補償金として弐億参千四百万円を出す事。尚、十一月三十日迄に貴社より回答ある事要求します。

昭和三十四年十一月二十五日

水俣病家庭互助会長
渡辺　栄蔵

新日窒水俣工場長
西田　栄一　殿

1959（昭和34）年12月1日　西日本新聞

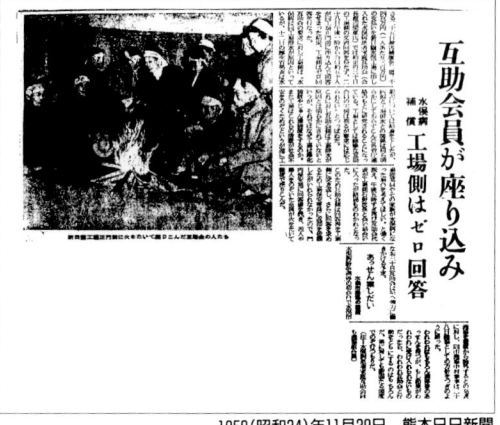

1959（昭和34）年11月29日　熊本日日新聞

「奇病・ヨイヨイ病」などと呼ばれ、隠れるように暮していた患者たちは、1959（昭和34）年にやっとチッソへ補償を要求して立上った。しかし患者を応援する人もなく、チッソ城下町の水俣でチッソに補償要求することは、町全体からつまはじきにされる覚悟が必要だった。

患者をだましたチッソ契約
―― 1959(昭和34)年 ――

（見舞金）契約書

第四条 甲(チッソ)は将来水俣病が甲(チッソ)の工場排水に起因しないことが決定した場合においてはその月をもって見舞金の交付は打ち切るものとする。

第五条 乙(患者)は将来、水俣病が甲(チッソ)の工場排水に起因することが決定した場合においても新たな補償金の要求は一切行なわないものとする。

チッソは、工場の廃水が原因で水俣病が発生することを知りながら、人を殺した償いとしてでなく「貧しい人へのお見舞い」として処理してしまった。それは、死者に30万円、生存者年金成人10万円、子供1万円という低額なものだった。 この 見舞金契約はのちの水俣病裁判で公序良俗に反するとして無効とされた。患者側に「工場が原因とわかっても新たな補償はしない」とも約束させている。

患者運動高揚期

新潟水俣病の発見を契機に、政府は、水俣病を初めて「チッソによる公害」と認める。チッソへの補償要求をめぐって、患者互助会は分裂し、一部は裁判に踏み切った。反公害の世論を背景に、活発な患者運動が展開された。また、新たに認定を得た患者は、チッソとの長期にわたる自主交渉を開始する。勝訴判決と患者自らの実力行動によって補償協定が締結されて、以後、認定された患者には補償金が支払われることとなった。

水俣病裁判判決
理　由　要　旨

「化学工場が、廃水を工場外に放流するにあたっては、常に最高の知識と技術を用いて廃水中に危険物混入の有無および動植物や人体に対する影響のいかんにつき調査研究を尽くして、その安全性を確認するとともに、万一有害であることが判明し、あるいはその安全性に疑念を生じた場合には直ちに操業を中止するなどして必要最大限の防止措置を講じ、とくに地域住民の生命・健康に対する危害を未然に防止すべき高度の注意義務を有するものといわなければならない。

いかなる工場といえども、地域住民の生命・健康を侵害し、これを犠牲にすることは許されないからである。」

「被告工場における廃水の水質が、法令上の制限基準や行政基準に合致し、その廃水処理方法が同業他事業所のそれより優れていたとしても、被告工場がアセト・アルデヒド廃水を放流した行為については、終始過失があったと推認するに十分であり、廃水の放流が、被告の企業活動そのものとしてなされたという意味において、被告は過失の責任を免れないものといわなければならない。」

「被告の利潤優先・人命軽視の基本姿勢こそ水俣病を発生させた根本原因である。」

　　　　　　　　　　　　　　　　　　　　熊本地方裁判所
　　　　　　　　　　　　　　　　　　　　1973年3月20日

協定書
—1973(昭和48)年—

協定書

水俣病患者東京本社交渉団と、チッソ株式会社とは、水俣病患者、家族に対する補償などの解決にあたり、次のとおり協定する。

〈前文〉

一、チッソ株式会社は、水俣工場で有害物質を含む排水を流し続け、廃棄物の処理を怠り、広く対岸の天草を含む水俣周辺海域を汚染してきた。その結果、悲惨な「水俣病」を発生させ、人間破壊をもたらしてきた事実を率直に認める。

昭和三十一年の水俣病公式発見後も、被害の拡大防止、原因究明、被害者救済等を行わなかったため、いよいよ被害を拡大させることとなったこと、及び原因物質が確認されるに至っても、問題が社会化するに及んでも、解決に遺憾な態度をとってきた経過についてチッソ株式会社は心から反省する。

しかも、チッソ株式会社及びその家族の水俣病による苦痛、苦しみ、貧窮にあえぐ患者及びその家族による苦痛、地域社会からの差別等により受けてきた経過に加えて種々の屈辱、地域社会からの差別等により受けてきた経過にチッソ株式会社は心から陳謝する。

二、チッソ株式会社は、解決を長びかせたことにより、社会に多大の迷惑をかけたこと、第三の水俣病問題で全国民が不安の状態にある今日、あらためて社会に対し深く謝罪する。

三、熊本地方裁判所は、チッソ株式会社の工場排水に起因したものであり、かつ、チッソ株式会社に過失責任ありとの原告の請求を全面的に認める「水俣病」判決を行なった。この判決に全面的に服し、その内容のすべてを誠実に履行する。

四、見舞金契約の締結等により水俣病にかかわった患者らを見舞金契約の締結等により水俣病にかかわった患者らを社会的に葬ったと言われても不知火海全域に患者がいることを認識せず、第三の水俣病の被害発見のための努力を怠り、現在に至るも水俣病の被害の深さや広さについてつくされていない事態をもたらしたのであり、これらは潜在患者に対する責任を全うしていないものである。チッソ株式会社は、この判決に全面的に服し、患者の救済のすべてに全力をあげることを約束する。

五、チッソ株式会社は、過去をふりかえる意味でも、今後、公害を絶対に発生させないため、具体的な方策と公害防止対策に全力を挙げて取り組む。現在汚染されている水俣周辺海域の浄化対策、これまでの排水の実情、関係資料等の提示を行ない、関係官庁、地方自治体、公害防止協定を早急に締結する。また、現在汚染されている水俣周辺海域の浄化対策、地方自治体、関係地方公共団体と公害防止協定を早急に締結する。

六、チッソ株式会社は、水俣病患者とその周辺に与えた迷惑はもとより、住民の不安を常に確認するとともに、関係地域に対する住民の不安を常に解消することに努める。

七、チッソ株式会社は、水俣病患者の治療及び訓練、社会復帰、職業あっせんその他の患者の福祉の増進について実情に即した具体的方策を誠意をもって講じて早急に具体的方策を誠意をもって講じて早急に実施する。

八、事態を紛糾せしめ、水俣病患者東京本社交渉団と交渉を続けてきたが、今日まで解決が遅延したことについて患者に遺憾の意を表する。

補償の現状

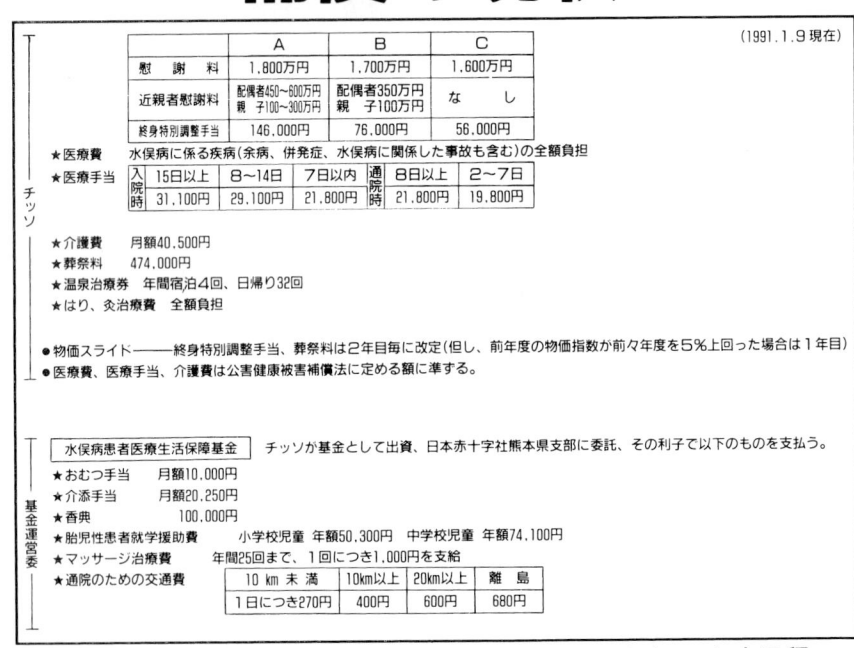

(1991.1.9現在)

		A	B	C
チッソ	慰謝料	1,800万円	1,700万円	1,600万円
	近親者慰謝料	配偶者450〜600万円 親 子100〜300万円	配偶者350万円 親 子100万円	なし
	終身特別調整手当	146,000円	76,000円	56,000円

★医療費　水俣病に係る疾病(余病、併発症、水俣病に関係した事故も含む)の全額負担

★医療手当

	入院時			通院時	
	15日以上	8〜14日	7日以内	8日以上	2〜7日
	31,100円	29,100円	21,800円	21,800円	19,800円

★介護費　月額40,500円
★葬祭料　474,000円
★温泉治療券　年間宿泊4回、日帰り32回
★はり、灸治療費　全額負担

● 物価スライド——終身特別調整手当、葬祭料は2年目毎に改定(但し、前年度の物価指数が前々年度を5%上回った場合は1年目)
● 医療費、医療手当、介護費は公害健康被害補償法に定める額に準する。

水俣病患者医療生活保障基金　チッソが基金として出資、日本赤十字社熊本県支部に委託、その利子で以下のものを支払う。

★おむつ手当　月額10,000円
★介添手当　月額20,250円
★香典　100,000円
★胎児性患者就学援助費　小学校児童 年額50,300円　中学校児童 年額74,100円
★マッサージ治療費　年間25回まで、1回につき1,000円を支給
★通院のための交通費

10 km 未満	10km以上	20km以上	離島
1日につき270円	400円	600円	680円

裁判や自主交渉といった長い闘いの中から、ようやくチッソにある程度の補償をさせることができた。約束は1973(昭和48)年7月9日に結ばれた。この協定書によって、チッソは認定された患者に補償を続けている。

社長との直接交渉

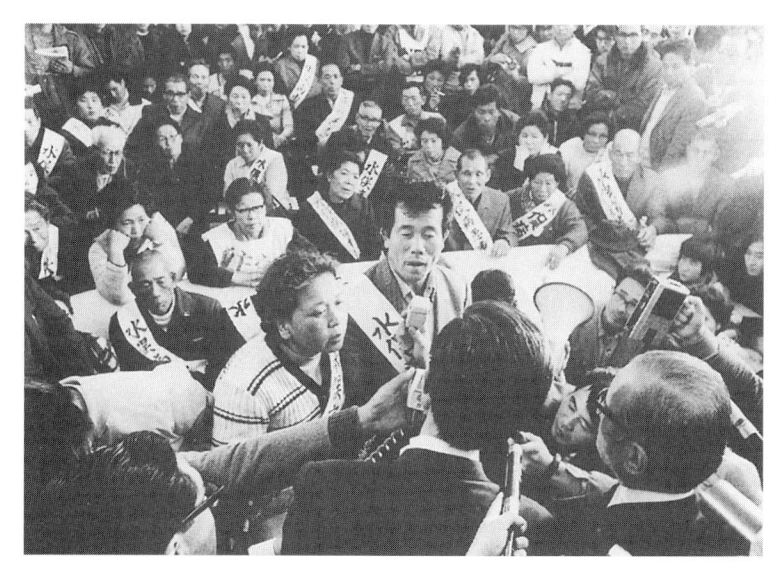

撮影　宮本成美　1973年

裁判を続けていた患者と、チッソの前に坐り込みを続けていた患者は、合同して「東京本社交渉団」を結成し、チッソとの交渉を開始した。

自主交渉坐り込み

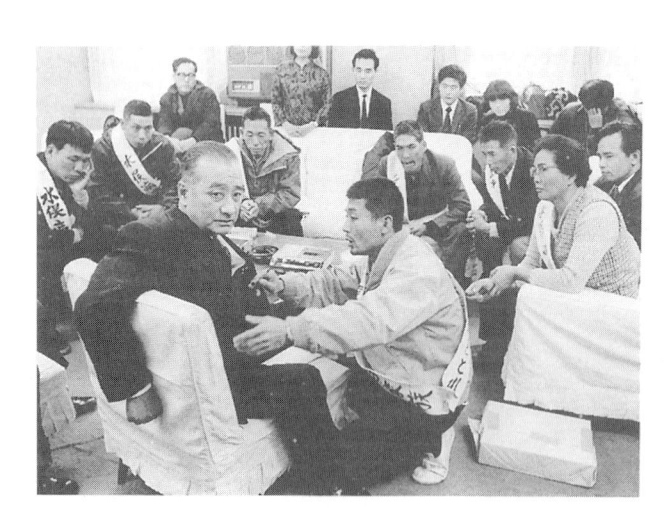

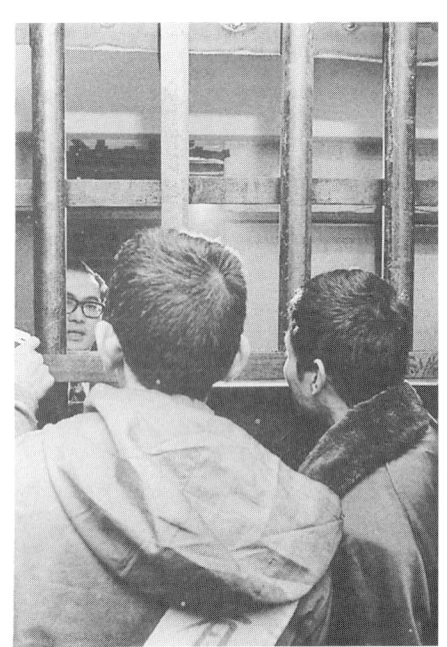

撮影　宮本成美　1973年

　熊本県から「水俣病ではない」と棄却されたことを、不服として、数人の患者が環境庁へ行政不服申立てを行った。環境庁は患者の主張を認め、「否定しえない者は、認定せよ」と熊本県に命令を下した。こうして示されたいわゆる「昭和46年環境庁裁決」によって認定された水俣病患者を、チッソは「前の認定患者とは違う」と補償交渉を拒否した。このため川本輝夫ら数人はチッソとの直接交渉を求め、坐り込みを続けた。「人の命に何の違いもない」として要求した一律3,000万円の補償要求に、水俣市民の多くは冷たい態度だった。

支援活動

水俣病患者のための支援活動は、長い間存在しなかったが、水俣病患者が裁判を始めた前後から、水俣市民有志による患者支援団体「水俣病市民会議」が作られた。「チッソの城下町・水俣」の中で、チッソにはむかう患者を支援することもまた決意が必要だった。こうした動きに触発されて、熊本市に「水俣病を告発する会」が作られ、以後東京・大阪等全国各地で、学生運動を経験した無党派の市民や文化人などを中心に同様の支援団体が生まれ、裁判や直接交渉の応援、援農援漁、患者運動の資金集めに動いてゆく。石牟礼道子の『苦海浄土』や土本典昭の映画『水俣——患者さんとその世界』等によって支援運動に加わるようになった者も少なくない。また水俣病弁護団によって弁護活動がはじめられた二次訴訟や三次訴訟は、革新政党や労働組合などからの支援によって支えられている。

認定制度への闘い

水俣病裁判の進行や第三水俣病などにより、水俣病問題が社会的に注目をされ、認定申請が続出するようになった。こうした事態に行政による認定業務は患者を認定しない方向で機能しはじめる。これに対して、未認定患者たちは、数々の裁判や直接交渉をもって、早く、広く認定することを求め続けた。裁判はすべて患者側の勝訴に終始するものの、環境庁や熊本県は判決に服することなく、近年にいたって認定制度は、患者を切り捨てるための制度としてその「威力」を発揮している。行政に失望した患者は再び加害者チッソに向かいはじめた。

認定・補償の仕組み

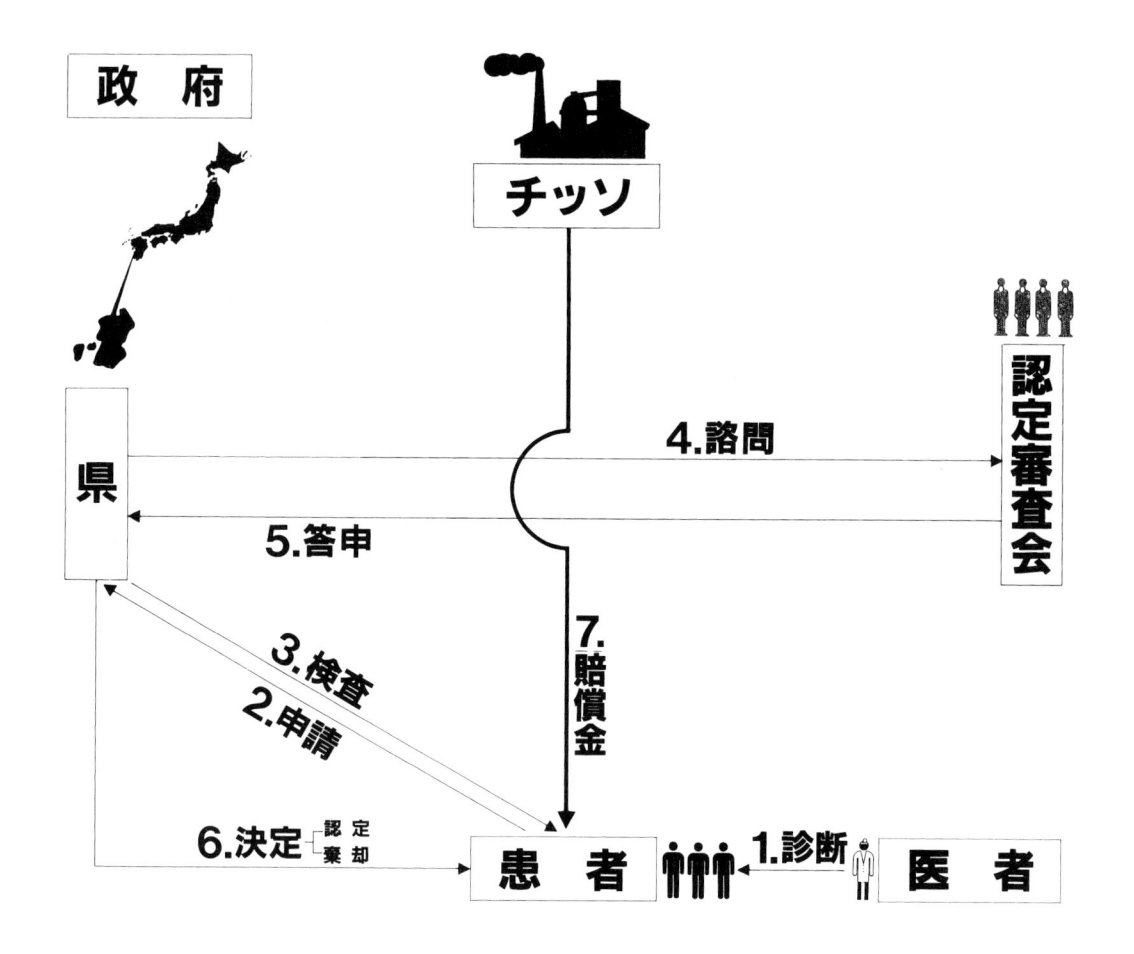

水俣病患者がチッソからの補償金を手に入れるためには、行政により被害者として「認定」されることが、その前提となっている。不知火海沿岸の汚染指定地区に居住し、水俣病の症状を持つ者は、医師の診断書を添付して県知事に認定申請する。県は申請者の検診を実施し、その記録を添えて、医師による認定審査会に諮問する。その答申を受けて、県知事は、認定か棄却かの処分を決定する。しかし運用の実態は、この制度を定めている「公害健康被害補償法」に照らしても、また、水俣病患者の置かれている現状から見ても、たいへん問題が多いことが指摘されている。

認定申請そのものが困難

調査 富樫貞夫・丸山定巳(熊本大学)1981年

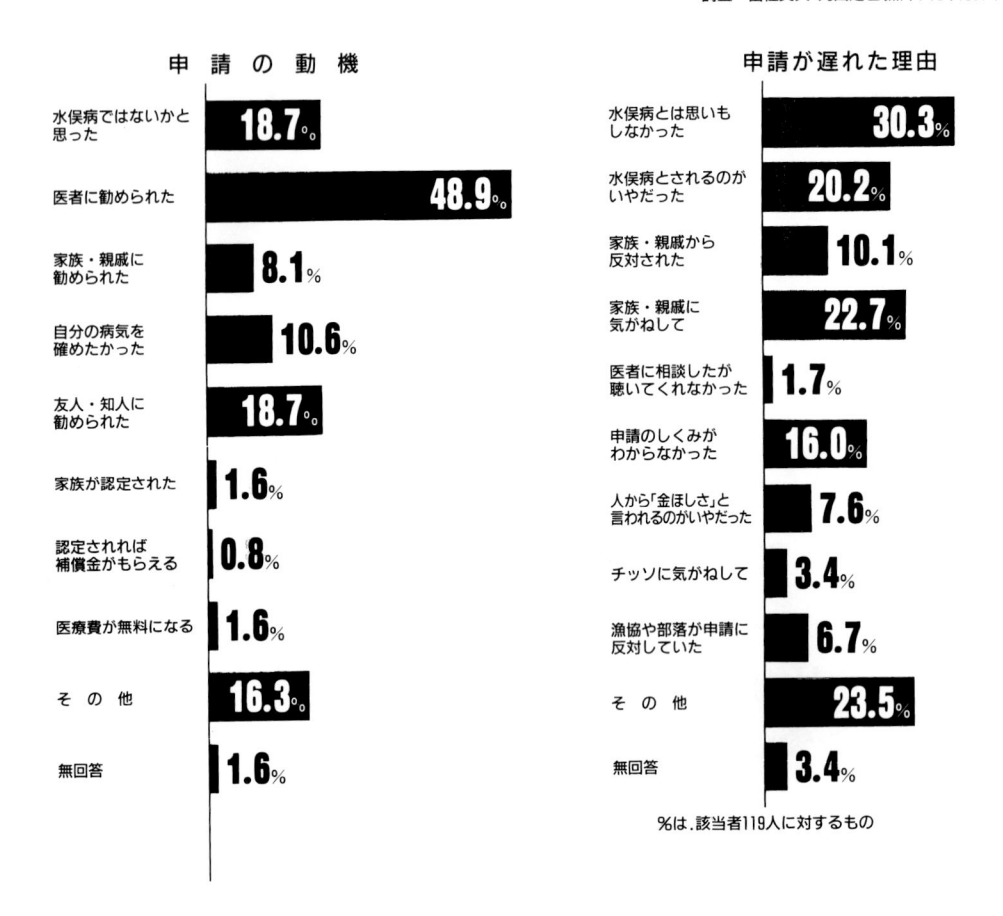

申請の動機

- 水俣病ではないかと思った　18.7%
- 医者に勧められた　48.9%
- 家族・親戚に勧められた　8.1%
- 自分の病気を確めたかった　10.6%
- 友人・知人に勧められた　18.7%
- 家族が認定された　1.6%
- 認定されれば補償金がもらえる　0.8%
- 医療費が無料になる　1.6%
- その他　16.3%
- 無回答　1.6%

申請が遅れた理由

- 水俣病とは思いもしなかった　30.3%
- 水俣病とされるのがいやだった　20.2%
- 家族・親戚から反対された　10.1%
- 家族・親戚に気がねして　22.7%
- 医者に相談したが聴いてくれなかった　1.7%
- 申請のしくみがわからなかった　16.0%
- 人から「金ほしさ」と言われるのがいやだった　7.6%
- チッソに気がねして　3.4%
- 漁協や部落が申請に反対していた　6.7%
- その他　23.5%
- 無回答　3.4%

%は、該当者119人に対するもの

申請も簡単なことではない。「水俣病患者や家族とは結婚しない」「そんなに金が欲しいのか」などと言われることを恐れ、申請しない人も多い。本人が申請しなければ、どんなに具合が悪くなっても、チッソは何もしない。国や県は、申請の方法を知らせる努力もしていない。魚は食べたが「まさか自分の具合の悪いのが水俣病だとは思わなかった」という人も多い。

申請しても切りすてられる

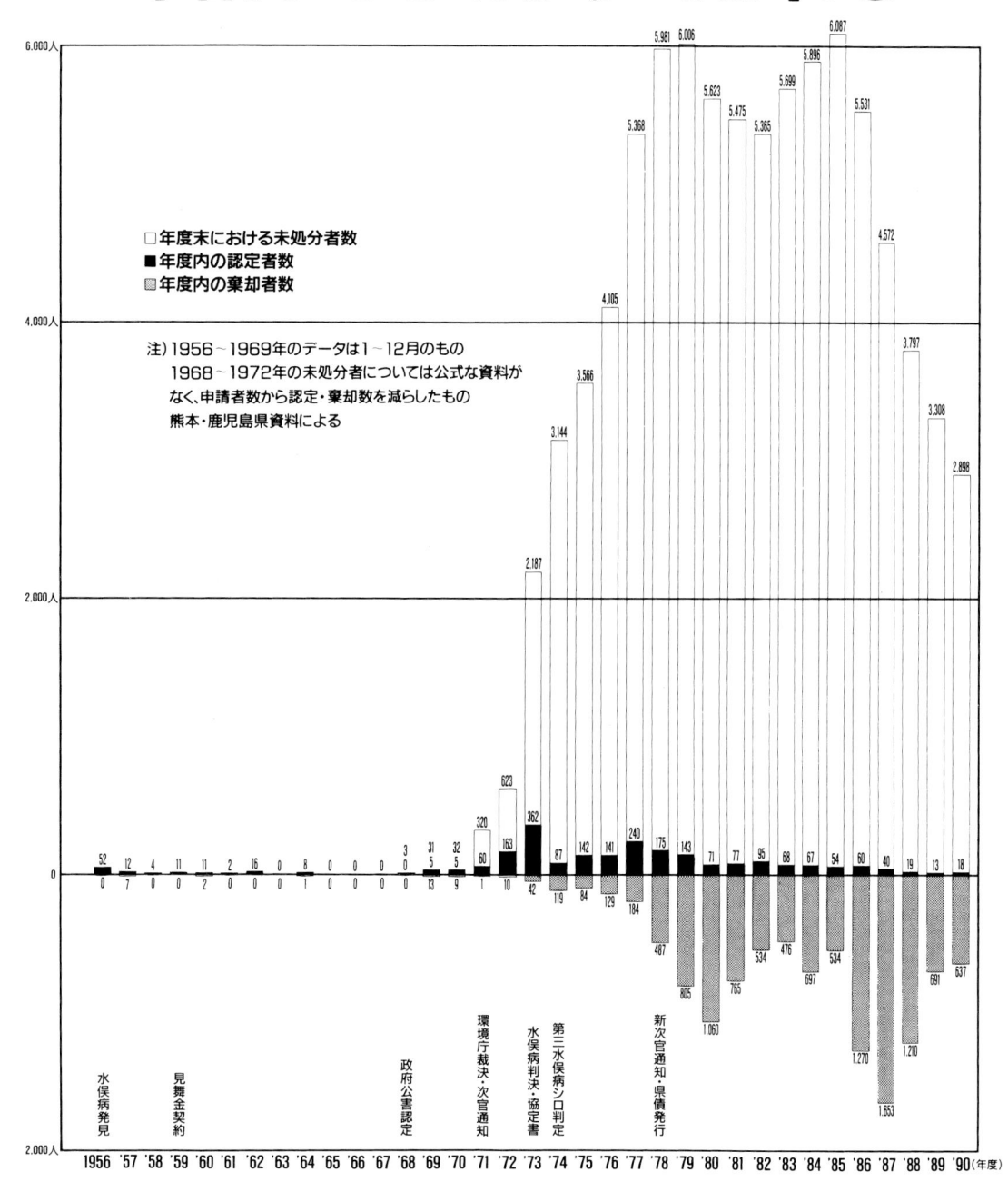

グラフ凡例:
- □ 年度末における未処分者数
- ■ 年度内の認定者数
- ▨ 年度内の棄却者数

注) 1956～1969年のデータは1～12月のもの
1968～1972年の未処分者については公式な資料がなく、申請者数から認定・棄却数を減らしたもの
熊本・鹿児島県資料による

年度	未処分者数	認定者数	棄却者数
1956		52	0
'57		12	7
'58		4	
'59		11	
'60		11	2
'61		2	
'62		16	
'63		0	
'64		8	
'65		0	
'66		0	
'67		3	0
'68		31	13
'69		5	9
'70		32	
'71		5	1
'72	320	60	10
'73	623	163	42
'74	2,187	362	119
'75	3,144	87	84
'76	3,566	142	129
'77	4,105	141	184
'78	5,368	240	487
'79	5,981	175	805
'80	6,006	143	1,060
'81	5,623	71	765
'82	5,475	77	534
'83	5,365	95	476
'84	5,699	68	697
'85	5,896	67	534
'86	6,087	54	1,270
'87	5,531	60	1,653
'88	4,572	40	1,210
'89	3,797	19	691
'90	3,308	13	637
	2,898	18	

年表（下段）:
- 水俣病発見
- 見舞金契約
- 政府公害認定
- 環境庁裁決・次官通知
- 水俣病判決・協定書
- 第三水俣病シロ判定
- 新次官通知・県債発行

水俣病の認定制度は「水俣病患者か否か」を判断するものとは言えず、「チッソが補償金を支払うべき対象か否か」を定めるためのものとして機能してきた。いわば、チッソの利益を守るための制度とさえ言える。行政によって「認定基準」は大きく変動し、1973年以降は大量に棄却される状態が続いている。切りすてられ、放置される被害者はあとをたたない。

これまでに認定された人びと

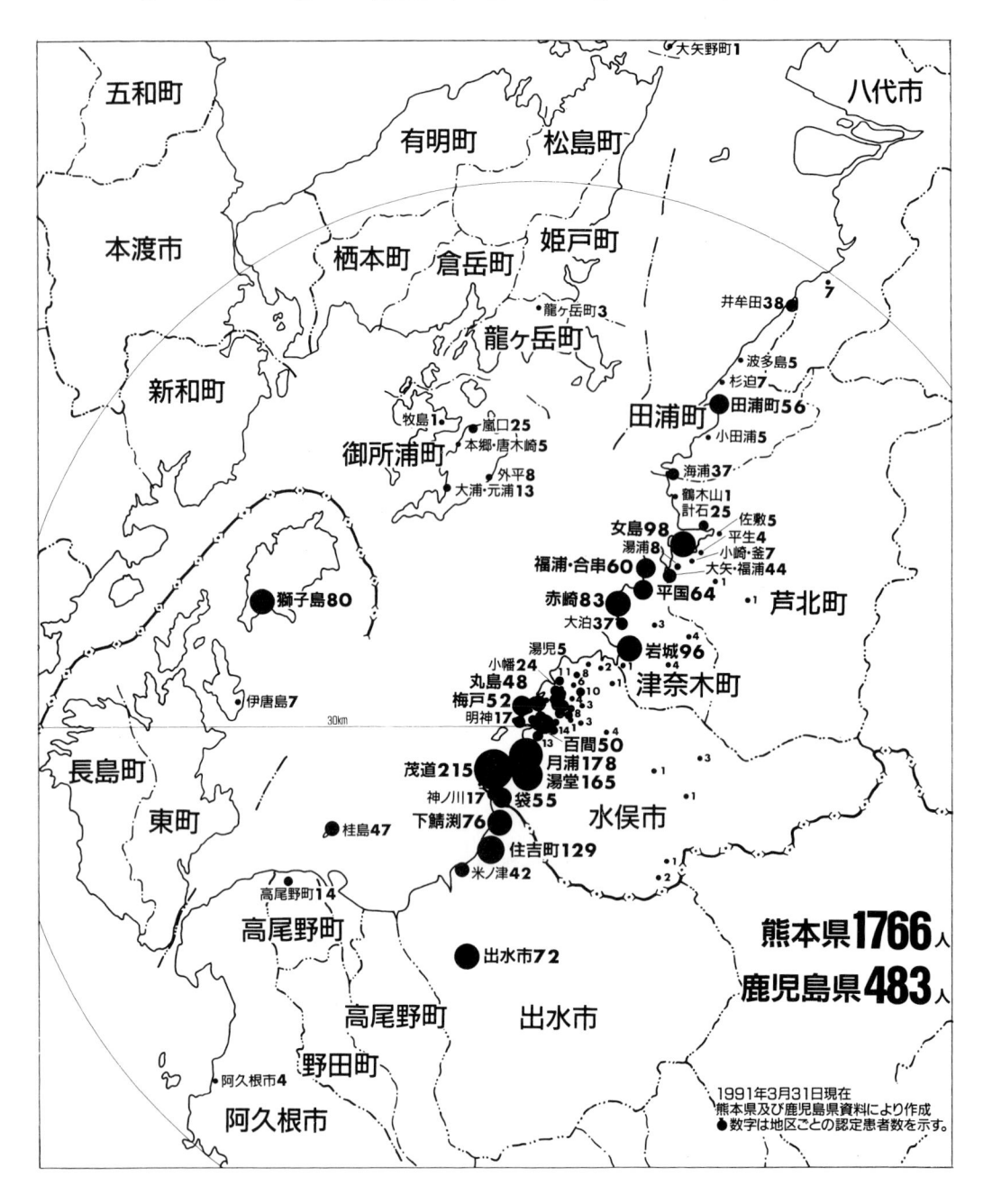

熊本県 **1766**人
鹿児島県 **483**人

1991年3月31日現在
熊本県及び鹿児島県資料により作成
● 数字は地区ごとの認定患者数を示す。

地図上の地名と認定患者数：
- 大矢野町 1
- 龍ヶ岳町 3
- 井牟田 38、7
- 牧島 1
- 嵐口 25
- 波多島 5
- 杉迫 7
- 本郷・唐木崎 5
- 田浦町 56
- 外平 8
- 小田浦 5
- 大浦・元浦 13
- 海浦 37
- 鶴木山 1
- 計石 25
- 佐敷 5
- 女島 98
- 平生 4
- 湯浦 8
- 小崎・釜 7
- 福浦・合串 60
- 大矢・福浦 44
- 赤崎 83
- 平国 64
- 大泊 37
- 岩城 96
- 湯児 5
- 小幡 24
- 丸島 48
- 津奈木町
- 梅戸 52
- 明神 17
- 百間 50
- 茂道 215
- 月浦 178
- 湯堂 165
- 神ノ川 17
- 袋 55
- 獅子島 80
- 伊唐島 7
- 桂島 47
- 下鯖渕 76
- 住吉町 129
- 米ノ津 42
- 高尾野町 14
- 出水市 72
- 阿久根市 4

有機水銀流出当時、不知火海沿岸には約30万人の人びとが暮らしていたことから、何らかの健康被害をうけた人びとは数万人に及ぶともいわれている。こうした人びとのうち、認定され補償金を受けとることが出来た人は、ほんの一部にすぎない。発病しながら、その原因も知らず死んでしまった人たちの数は、永久に明らかにはならない。

現在──私たちの課題
4

水俣湾のヘドロ処理

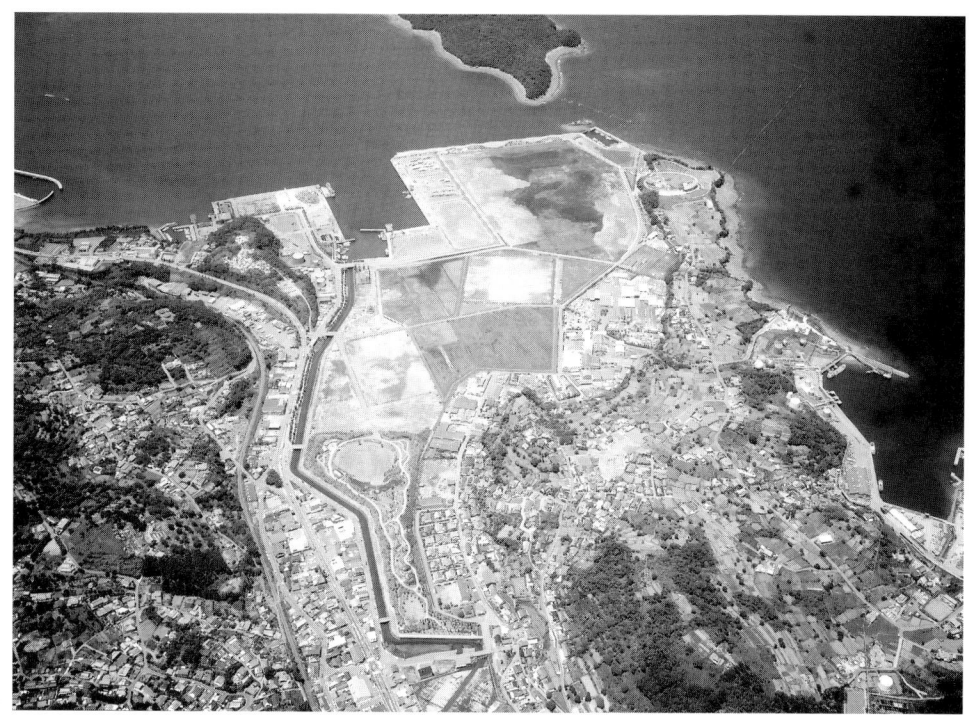

水俣湾埋立地

　チッソが36年間にわたって流し続けた水銀は水俣湾内外にヘドロと共に堆積した。熊本県は1977年から総事業費485億円と約13年の年月をかけて、湾内の水銀濃度25PPM以上のヘドロ約151万立方メートルを一部浚渫、一部埋め立てにより処理した。その結果、水俣湾に水銀ヘドロと汚染魚を封じ込めた約58ヘクタールの埋立地が出現した。
　しかし、このヘドロ処理工事による湾外へのヘドロ拡散と二次汚染が懸念された。そのため患者や住民が工事差し止めの裁判を起こしたが敗訴した。また、環境庁による暫定除去基準の算出方法に疑問が持たれた。水俣湾の処理基準は25PPMであったが、山口県徳山湾の場合は、10PPMであった。この違いについて住民に納得のいく説明はなされなかった。
　ヘドロ処理によって水銀が消えたわけではない。今後も湾内に残る水銀や埋立地に沈められた水銀の監視を続けなければならない。一度環境汚染を引き起こしてしまえば、人間は汚染物質と果てしなくつき合っていくしかない。その例が水俣湾埋立地である。

水俣湾の仕切網と魚介類の現状

仕切網は、水銀値の高い魚が市場に出回るのではないかという熊本県民の不安解消と県内他海域の魚価の安定のために、1974年に熊本県によって水俣湾口に設置された。湾内の魚介類は、チッソが買い上げ、焼却処分した。その後、チッソからの水銀排出が1968年に止まったことと、ヘドロ処理により、湾内の魚介類の水銀値は下がり、厚生省の定めた暫定規制値を下回った。しかし、1997年までは水俣湾の魚介類の漁獲、販売、摂取は自粛されていた。熊本県は1魚種に付き10検体の平均値を採用しているが、単体では暫定規制値を越える魚がいた。この暫定規制値の総水銀0.4PPM、メチル水銀0.3PPMは、魚介類の平均最大摂取量を1日108.9gとして定められたもので、1日1kg食べることもまれではない不知火海沿岸漁民の食生活が考慮されていない。また、総水銀のほとんどがメチル水銀であるという研究もある。

1997年10月、仕切り網は水俣湾内の魚介類の平均水銀値が暫定規制値を下回ったため、撤去された。水俣病の教訓を活かし、水俣湾の魚介類の安全性を確認するためには、専門家や行政のみに任せるのではなく、被害者や住民が自ら論議することが求められている。

仕切網の変遷

設置期間	設置期間等	網の位置・構造
1974年1月10日 ～1975年8月20日 期間約1年9カ月	熊本県水産課 （1975年4月1日から 熊本県公害部） 仕切網延長 2,350m	
1975年8月21日 ～1977年9月30日 期間約2年1カ月	熊本県環境公害部 仕切網延長 1,550m （全長2,200m）	
1977年10月1日 ～1993年9月30日 期間16年	熊本県環境公害部 （1990年4月1日から チッソ株式会社） 仕切網延長 3,662m （全長7,495m）	
1993年10月1日 ～1995年6月30日 期間1年8カ月	チッソ株式会社 仕切網延長 4,404m （内仕切網742mを含む）	
1995年7月1日 ～1997年10月14日 期間約2年3カ月	チッソ株式会社 仕切網延長 2,106m	

（注） この図は、熊本県環境公害部の資料に基づいて作成した。

水俣湾内の魚介類の水銀値と仕切網

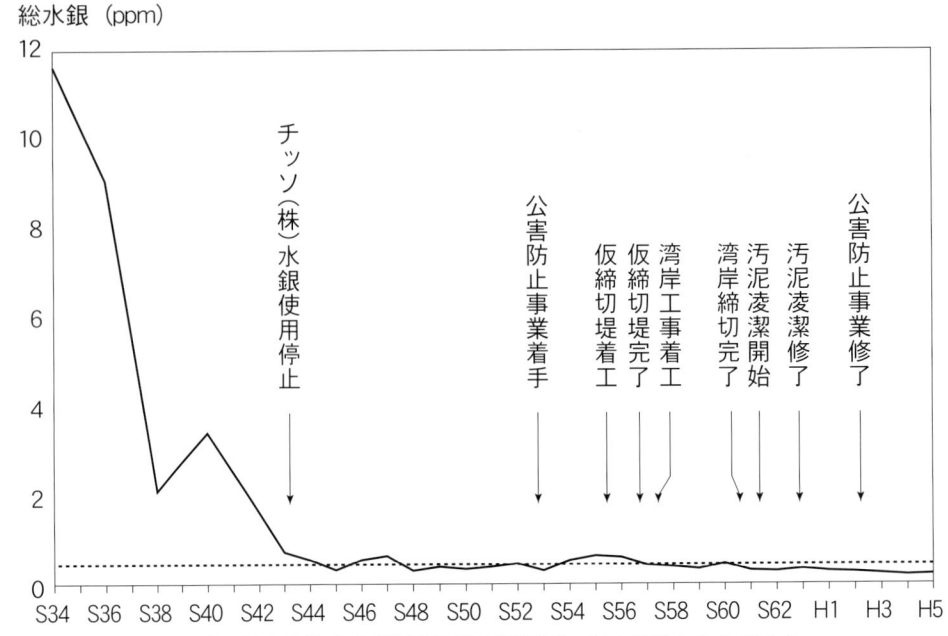

総水銀（ppm）

グラフ中の注記（縦書き矢印ラベル、左から右）：
- チッソ（株）水銀使用停止
- 公害防止事業着手
- 湾岸工事着工
- 仮締切堤着工
- 仮締切堤着完了
- 湾岸締切完了
- 汚泥浚渫開始
- 汚泥浚渫修了
- 公害防止事業修了

横軸：S34 S36 S38 S40 S42 S44 S46 S48 S50 S52 S54 S56 S58 S60 S62 H1 H3 H5

（注）
1 グラフ中の総水銀値は、各種調査結果を調査年次ごとに平均したものです。
2 グラフ中の波線は、国が定めた魚介類の水銀の暫定規制値（総水銀：0.4ppm）を示す。
3 グラフは、熊本県環境公害部環境総務課が編集した。

熊本県による水俣湾の魚類調査結果 （単位ppm）

魚種	1974-75年 平均値 最低一最高	1989年 平均値 最低一最高	1992年 平均値 最低一最高	1994年 平均値 最低一最高	1995年 平均値 最低一最高	1996年 平均値 最低一最高
アカエイ	0.876 0.17-1.49	0.47 0.15-0.78	0.89 0.45-1.11	0.30 0.12-0.64	0.24 0.10-0.38	0.24 0.12-0.42
シロギス	1.030 0.62-1.40	1.04 0.46-1.87	0.79 0.57-1.22	0.39 0.20-0.52	0.31 0.19-0.54	0.28 0.16-0.51
アイナメ	―	0.98 0.30-1.36	0.70 0.30-1.13	0.33 0.23-0.52	―	―
シマイサキ		0.96	0.68	0.32 0.18-0.49		
カサゴ	0.845 0.42-1.73	0.68 0.51-1.02	0.53 0.39-0.62	0.31 0.20-0.43	0.29 0.25-0.36	0.24 0.16-0.36
クロダイ	0.121 0.06-0.33	0.63 0.11-1.63	0.26 0.06-0.82	0.20 0.07-0.29	0.13 0.09-0.23	0.13 0.07-0.26
ササノハベラ	0.514 0.34-0.77	0.40 0.33-0.62	0.25 0.20-0.30	0.20 0.15-0.25	0.20 0.16-0.23	0.13 0.08-0.17
スズキ	0.269 0.14-0.80	0.27 0.16-0.71	0.07 0.05-0.10	0.10 0.05-0.15	0.11 0.08-0.15	0.10 0.08-0.11

（注）1 熊本県の調査方法は、1魚種につき150グラムの資料を1検体として作成している。10検体の水銀の平均を平均値とし、最低・最高は調査した検体の数値である。
2 この表に示された数字は総水銀の値である。
3 1989～1995年のデータはその年度の後期調査のものであり、1996年は96年度前期調査のものを使用している。データは全て熊本県の調査によるものである。

チッソ貸付資金のしくみ

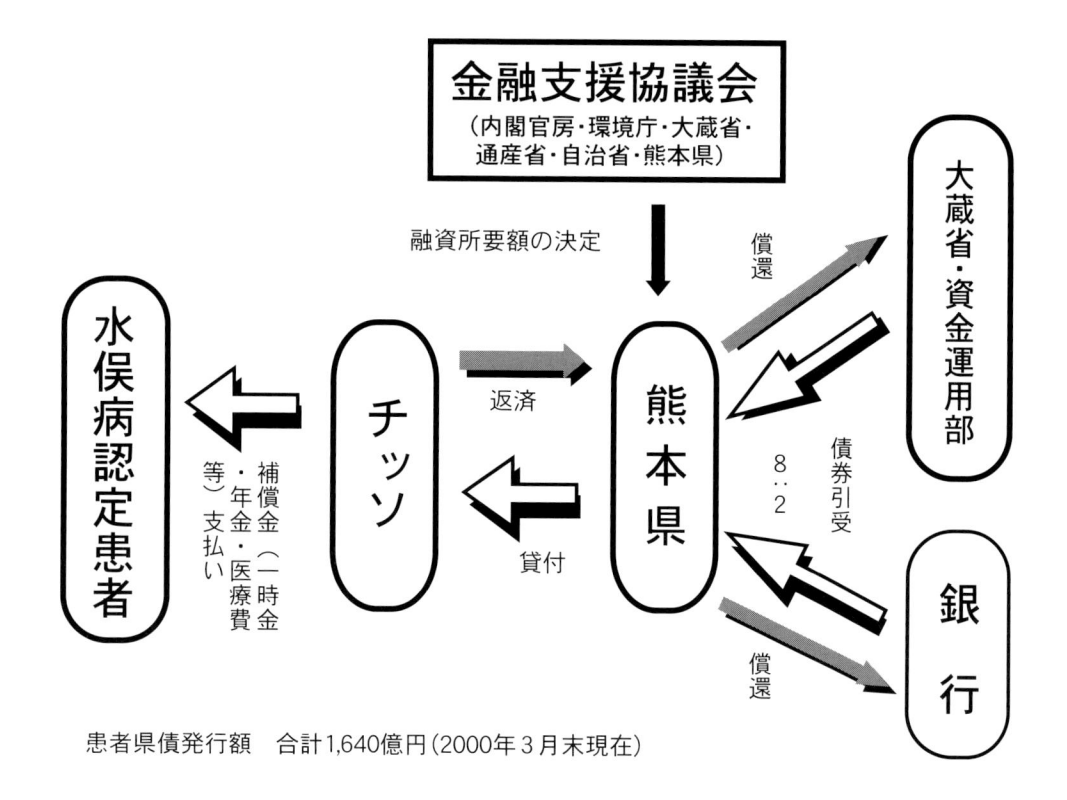

```
          金融支援協議会
       (内閣官房・環境庁・大蔵省・
        通産省・自治省・熊本県)
                │
      融資所要額の決定         償還        大蔵省・資金運用部
                ↓         ↗
   水俣病認定患者 ← チッソ → 熊本県 ⇄ 債券引受 8:2
          補償金(一時金  返済      ↑↓
          ・年金・医療            貸付  償還
          費等)支払い                    銀行
```

患者県債発行額　合計1,640億円(2000年3月末現在)

チッソ県債の種類と発行額

県債の種類	金額（利子を含む） （2000年3月現在）	目的・備考
患者県債	約1,640億円	認定患者への補償金の支払い。
ヘドロ県債	約688億円	水俣湾水銀ヘドロ処理・埋め立て工事費用
設備県債	約120億円	チッソ経営建て直しのための設備投資資金
一時金県債	約120億円	政府解決策による未認定患への一時金支払い （2000年3月31日貸付金の85％相当額を償還免除後）
合計	約2,568億円	

チッソに患者補償を滞りなく行わせるため、熊本県は1978年から県債を発行している。利子の総額は元金を上回っており、チッソの負債は増える一方である。

チッソの経営状況

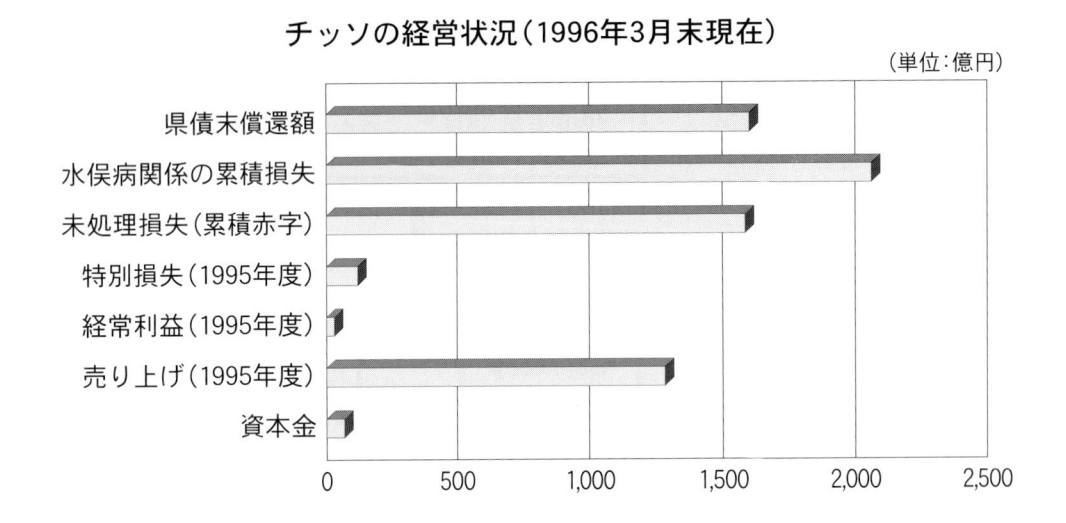

チッソの経営状況（1996年3月末現在）

（単位：億円）

県債末償還額	約1,600
水俣病関係の累積損失	約2,050
未処理損失（累積赤字）	約1,600
特別損失（1995年度）	わずか
経常利益（1995年度）	わずか
売り上げ（1995年度）	約1,300
資本金	わずか

チッソの累積赤字は資本金の20倍以上（1996年3月現在）にも上がっている。チッソは県債を償還するだけでも毎年80億円以上の支出が必要だと言われているが、1995年度の経営利益は31億円に過ぎない。

国と県の協力なしにはチッソは認定患者への補償すらできない。1978年以来、財政危機が続いているチッソが倒産しないのは行政が支えてきたからである。国や県がチッソを倒産させなかったのは、水俣病事件が大きな社会問題となっていたためである。社会問題化させた患者たちの運動が結果的にチッソの倒産を回避させてきた。一方では、行政が被害者救済や環境復元に深く係わらざるを得なかったことは行政にも責任があったことの証でもある。水俣病はチッソという一企業とそれを支えてきた国家政策によって作られた。公害が発生し健康と環境が破壊されれば一企業だけでは責任を果たすことはできない。

未認定患者の現状

1996年4月30日　水俣病患者連合とチッソとの「協定書」調印式

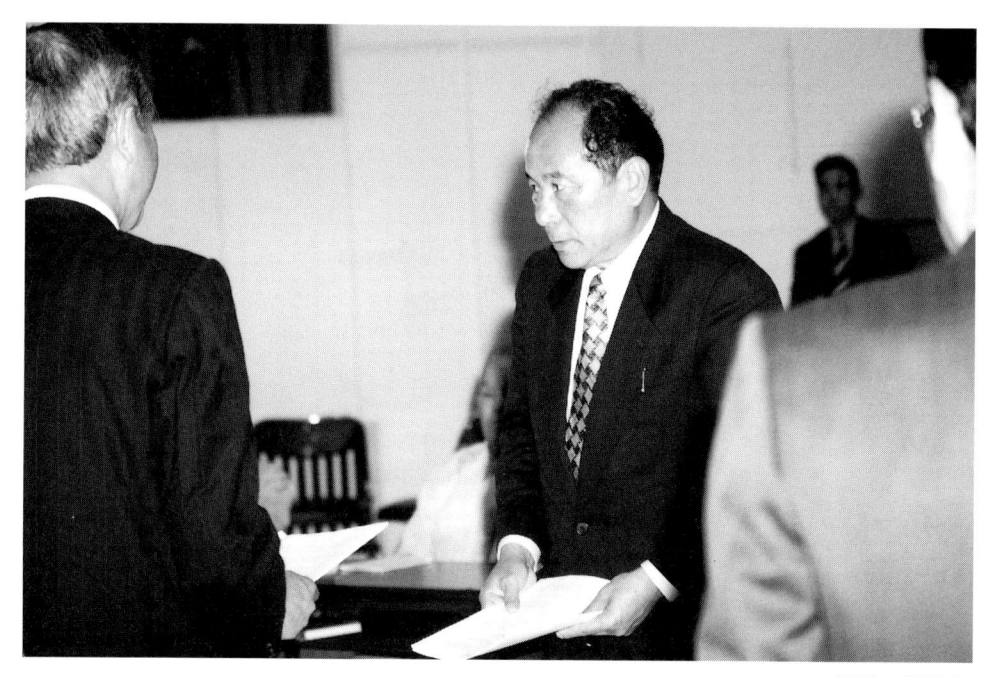

撮影　芥川 仁

1978年、政府はチッソへの金融支援を決定すると同時に認定基準を厳しくした。これにより認定制度は「患者切り捨て制度」へと変貌し、認定申請しても患者はほとんど認定されなくなった。未認定患者たちは、訴訟や自主交渉によって補償を求め運動を続けたが、政府の方針は変わらなかった。1995年、政府は最終解決案を提示した。高齢化し、残された力と時間が僅かしかなかったほとんどの患者団体はこれを受け入れざるを得なかった。こうして水俣病公式確認以来40年目にして患者補償問題はほぼ決着した。しかし、患者たちが強く求めていた「水俣病患者としての救済」「行政の責任を明らかにすること」は曖昧な形のまま置き去りにされた。これらを明確にしていくことは、水俣病事件を後世に生かすためにも必要であり、地域再生事業と共に今後に残された課題である。

政府解決案に伴うチッソ支援などのしくみ

1995年の政府解決策では、患者県債とは異なり、救済対象者への一時金の大部分を国家予算（一般会計・税金）から支出している。

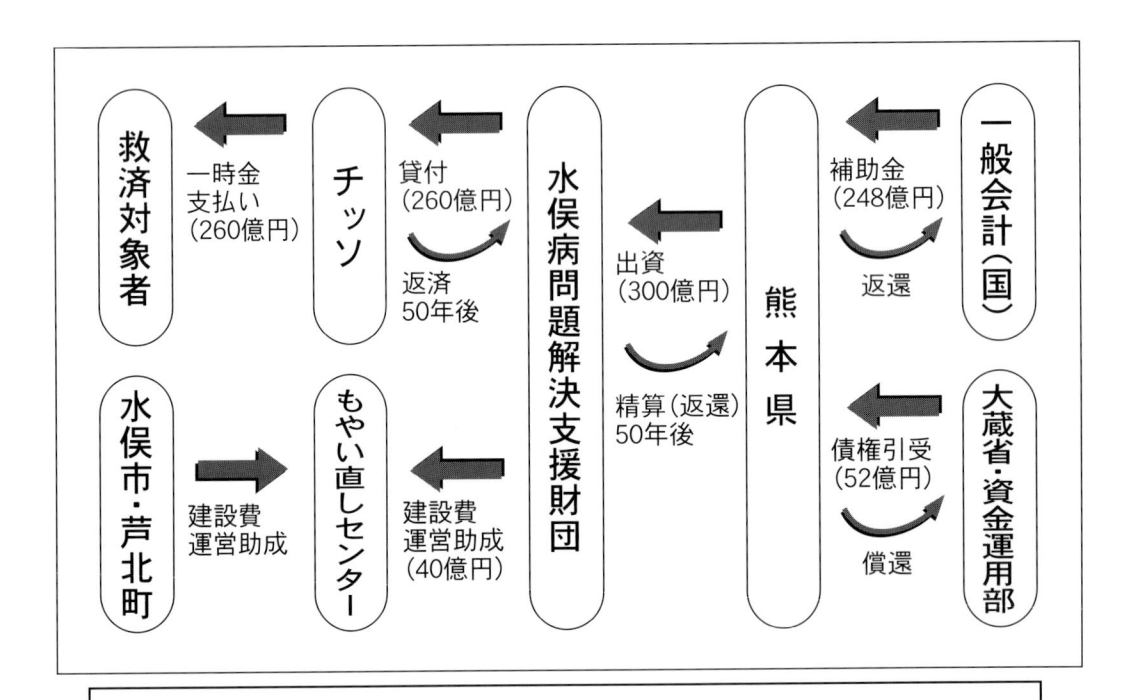

```
救済対象者 ← 一時金支払い(260億円) ← チッソ ← 貸付(260億円)/返済50年後 ← 水俣病問題解決支援財団 ← 出資(300億円)/精算(返還)50年後 ← 熊本県 ← 補助金(248億円)/返還 ← 一般会計(国)
                                                                                                                              熊本県 ← 債権引受(52億円)/償還 ← 大蔵省・資金運用部
水俣市・芦北町 → 建設費運営助成 → もやい直しセンター ← 建設費運営助成(40億円) ← 水俣病問題解決支援財団
```

政府解決策骨子

1、企業は、水俣病の原因となったメチル水銀を排出した者としての社会的債務を認識し、総合対策医療事業の対象者（判定検討会が認めた者を含む）に一時金を支払う
2、一時金の額は一人当たり260万円。5つの被害者団体に属するものは一定額を加算する
3、国と熊本県は遺憾の意など何らかの責任ある態度を表明する
4、救済を受ける者は損害賠償訴訟などを取り下げる
5、国・県はチッソ支援、地域再生・振興のための施策などに取り組む

解決策では未認定患者に対する補償と共に地域再生・振興がうたわれ、水俣・芦北にもやい直しセンターが作られた。

1994年7月11日水俣病関西訴訟の一審判決（大阪地裁）

国、県に行政責任なし

水俣病関西訴訟　大阪地裁判決

チッソに賠償命令

20年の時効で12人棄却

和解による解決要請

原告、控訴を検討
きょうチッソ、国と交渉

関係者談話
最悪の判決

（『熊本日日新聞』1994年7月12日）

国家賠償を求める訴訟の多くは和解によって終結した。しかし、不知火海沿岸から関西に移住した患者たちが、行政の責任と水俣病との認定、被害補償を求めて起こした裁判は続けられている。一審判決では原告の多くが被害補償を認められたが、行政の責任は否定された。

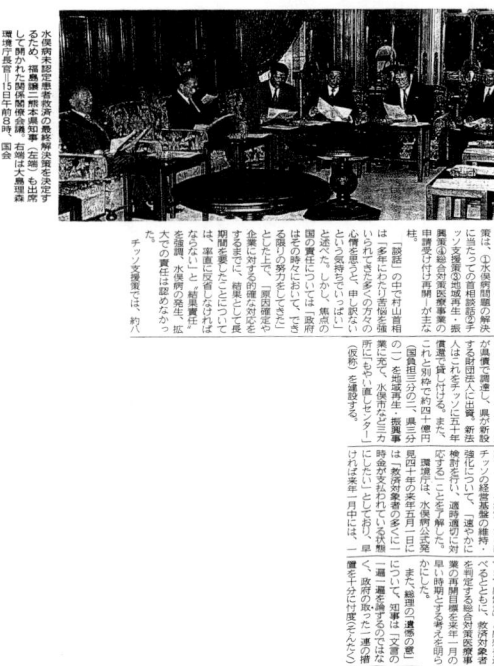

行政にも責任がある

「水俣病率直に反省」1996年12月16日『熊本日日新聞』

水俣病「率直に反省」
村山首相が談話

発生、拡大責任触れず

解決策が最終決定

未認定被害者 救済システム整う

1995年12月15日「水俣病問題の解決に当たっての内閣総理大臣談話抜粋」

解決に当たり、私は、苦しみと無念の思いの中でなくなられた方々に深い哀悼の念をささげますとともに、多年にわたり筆舌に尽くしがたい苦悩を強いられてこられた多くの方々の癒しがたい心情を思うとき、誠に申し訳ないという気持ちで一杯であります。水俣病の原因の確定や企業に対する的確な対応をするまでに、結果として長期間を要したことについて率直に反省しなければならないと思います。

国と熊本県には、水俣病の被害拡大と患者放棄の責任がある。水俣病被害の発生が確認された後も、チッソの廃水停止や漁獲禁止を行わず被害を拡大させた。また初期の段階で、不知火海沿岸住民の全面的な健康調査を実施せず、被害の拡がりを把握しなかった。さらに、救済を求める人々の訴えを、長く放置し続けた。国や県は「誠に申し訳ない気持ち」「遺憾に思う」などの表明を行うのみで、明確な謝罪は行わずいまだに責任を認めていない。

もやい直しの始まり

火のまつり

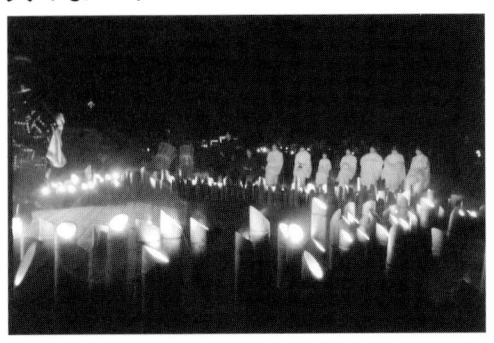

水俣病で失われた多くの命を想い、毎年水俣湾埋立地で行われている。

もやい直しセンター

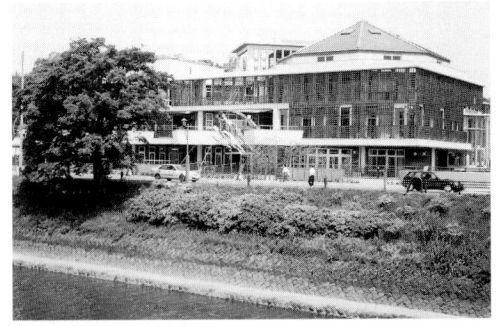

水俣病患者と地域住民の相互理解と新たな関係づくりのために作られた。

　患者たちとチッソの闘いは長く続いたが、チッソ企業城下町水俣の住民はそれを快くは思わなかった。患者と地域住民との間には対立が生まれ、いつしか越えがたい大きな壁となっていった。それは患者やチッソ関係者だけではなく、すべての地域住民、地元行政にとっても看過できない存在となっていった。

　水俣湾の埋め立てが終わった1990年から、熊本県と水俣市は「環境創造みなまた推進事業」を開始し、さまざまな事業が行われた。1995年には未認定患者補償問題にも一応の決着がつき、患者と市民や行政との関係は大きく変わった。そういった中で切れた絆を結び直そうと「もやい直し」の機運が患者、地域住民、地元行政の間で高まってきた。

　行政主催の市民講座で患者たちは自らの経験を語り始めた。水俣病で失われた命に祈る「火のまつり」は患者と行政との話し合いの中で生まれ、海・山・里の住民の協働によって続けられている。患者と地域住民がともに語り合い、新しい関係を作るための場として「もやい直しセンター」が建設された。

　しかし、長く続いてきた対立は一朝一夕に解消するものではない。地域・人・自然の再生は患者・地域住民・行政・チッソを含めたすべての関係者が取り組むべき課題である。それは困難な作業ではあるが、対立を創造のエネルギーに変えていくことによって初めてもやい直しは可能になるだろう。

水俣病を問い続ける

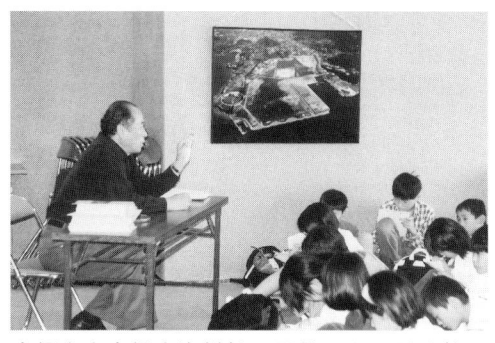

水俣市立水俣病資料館で子供たちに話す佐々木清澄さん。資料館には年間3万人が訪れる。

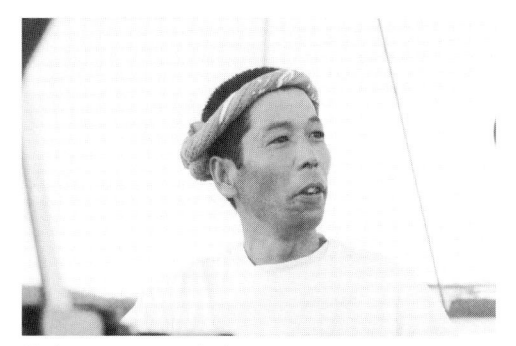

緒方正人さんは患者としてではなく人間として、水俣病を引き起こした人間の存在を問い続けている。

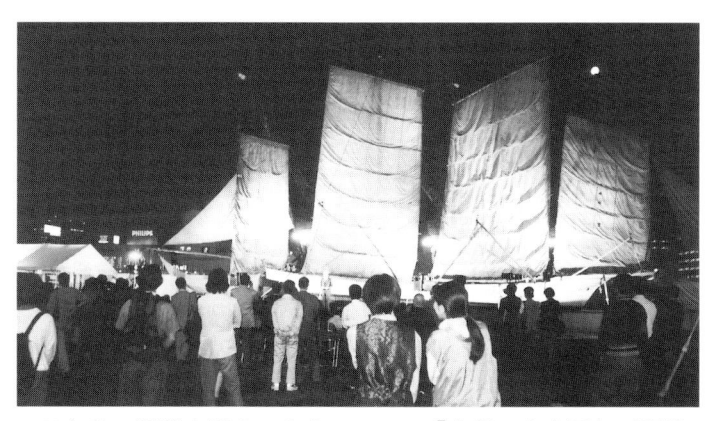

1996年秋、近代を問うことをテーマに「水俣・東京展」が開催され、3万人が集まった。

水俣病患者達はこれまで水俣や日本国内だけでなく、世界中に出かけ自らの体験を語り継いできた。しかし、水俣病発生から40年が経ち、患者たちは高齢化している。
現在、水俣では市立水俣病資料館や水俣病歴史考証館が水俣病事件の展示を行っている。また、相思社では水俣を訪れる人々に、水俣病理解のためにフィールドワーク、セミナーの開催、出版など様々なプログラムを提供している。
水俣病事件とは何であったのか。それを語り継ぐことができるのは、患者だけではない。水俣病に関わる人々がそれについて考え深化し、伝えようとする強い意思を持ち続けることが、水俣病の意味を明らかにしていくに違いない。

水俣病の教訓を生かすために

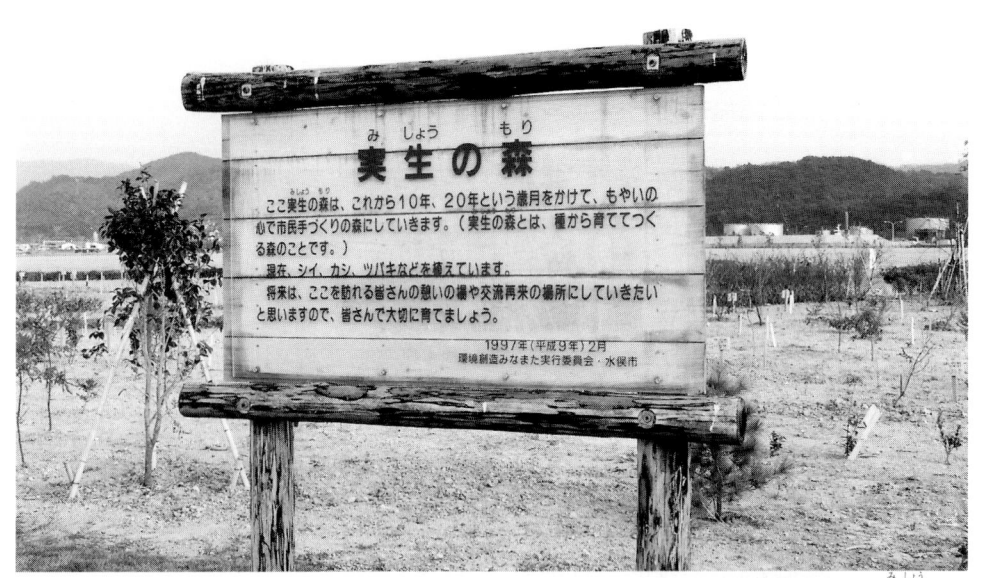

水俣湾埋立地の実生の森

1996年、水俣病の補償問題は一応の決着をみた。しかし、失われた命や健康、埋め立てられた海、そして海と共にあった生活は元通りになることはない。加害者を追及し、原因企業に責任を認めさせたのは、患者たちの闘いによるものだった。水俣病事件の歴史の中で企業や行政が自ら行動を起こし、償いをしたことはなかった。

20世紀は、技術革新によって様々なものが生み出された時代といえる。しかし、人間は自らを滅ぼす技術や物質まで生み出してしまった。水俣病は、日本という国が自然と人間のつながりを切り捨て、工業の発展による近代化を選択したときにあえて犯した失敗だった。人間は被害者にも加害者にもなる。水俣病の経験を被害者側からも加害者側からも包み隠さず伝えることは、水俣病に関わった者の、未来に対する責任ではないだろうか。

財団法人 水俣病センター相思社

■**財団法人水俣病センター相思社設立目的**
この法人は水俣病患者ならびに関係者の生活全般の問題について相談、解決にあずかるとともに、水俣病に関する調査、研究活動をおこなうことを目的とする。
　●設立／1974年4月7日
　●理事長／富樫貞夫（2002年11月1日現在）

■**相思社がめざすもの**
水俣病多発地から丘を少し登ったところに相思社があります。眼下には不知火海がゆったりとたたずんでいます。半世紀ほど前、不知火海に面した漁村に得体の知れない病気が発生しました。病に冒された人々は近隣の人々のさげすみの目を避けるようにひっそりと暮らしていました。なぜ、罪科のない人々が理不尽な苦しみを強いられなければならなかったのでしょうか。
水俣病事件は一企業の犯罪にはとどまりません。便利で豊かな生活を追い求めるという、ごく当たり前とされる行為が歴史の必然として産み落とした事件でした。水俣病患者は歴史の、人間の欲望の犠牲者だったのです。
半世紀を経た今も人々は便利さ・豊かさという呪縛から解き放たれてはいません。水俣病事件は人間のあり方を根元的に問い続けています。水俣病事件の真実と意味を明らかにすることは人類の未来にとって重要な意味があります。相思社はそのために努力を続けています。

■**利用案内**
相思社はこんなことに利用できます。
●水俣病学習・研修を目的とされる方の
　☆宿泊／20人程度まで・1人1泊1260円（要予約）食事は自炊になります。
　☆学習会・街案内／計画立案や費用のご相談など、お問い合わせ下さい。
　☆資料提供／資料室の利用ができます。事前にご連絡下さい。
●『ごんずい』（相思社機関紙）を年6回発行しています。水俣病事件の投げかけた意味をこれからの生き方に重ねあわせて考えていきます。購読料年間2100円。

水俣病歴史考証館

　水俣病事件は、現代社会を映す鏡です。企業活動による環境破壊と多数の犠牲者の発生、生活の糧である沿岸漁業の破壊、患者に対する偏見や差別、企業城下町での市民と患者との対立、市民もまた受けた外からの差別、このような被害を生み出すことをいわば原動力としながら日本は経済発展を遂げてきたのです。さらに、政治や行政のあり方、破壊された自然を回復することの難しさ、癒されない被害者の存在、人の痛みが見えない現代社会における人間疎外など、近代文明や人間社会が抱える様々な問題をも凝縮しています。

　私たちの暮らしを問いつづけ、今も動いている水俣病事件をテーマとする限り、考証館は、単なる過去の遺物の展示館ではありえません。絶えず、聞き取りやフィールドワークなどによって資料収集を行い、それを整理・研究し、そして考証館だけでなく、機関誌発行やセミナー開催、環境学習プログラムなどを通じて発信することが、総体として考証館活動なのだと考えています。

　このことは、来館者にとっては、水俣病事件の記憶を刻み込んだ地域全体が本当の博物館ということです。施設としての考証館は、患者の語りを聞く、自然に直に触れる、土地の暮らしを体験する、その入り口でありたいと思っています。

　「このままでは俺たちは犬死だ」という患者の言葉があります。考証館は、被害者の犠牲を無駄にせず、水俣病が起こらないような世の中にするため、水俣病を「記録し伝える」ことを続けます。

■水俣病歴史考証館

「不知火海―豊かな海と暮らし」「水俣病―チッソの犯罪」「闘い―被害者の道のり」「現在―私たちの課題」の4つのテーマから見た写真・解説パネル約100枚。木船、漁具、チッソ製品、工場内の道具、ネコ実験の小屋、チッソ社長詫び状、チッソ東京本社鉄格子、水銀ヘドロ、汚染魚、漁獲自粛看板、汚染魚仕切網、書字障害筆跡、患者手帳、ビラ合戦のチラシ、『苦海浄土』自筆原稿など実物多数。

　　　　休館日●年末年始　　開館時間●午前9時～午後5時
　　　　入館料●大人525円、高校生420円、小中学生315円
　　　　　　　20人以上の団体は105円引
　　　　　　※修学旅行など、多人数の見学についてはご相談ください。大型バスは進入で
　　　　　　　きませんので、駐車場をご案内します。

■維持会員のお願い

　相思社の活動は皆様からの維持会費や寄付によって支えられています。ご賛同・ご協力いただくこととともに、連帯の輪が広がることを願っています。口も手も出していただき、

水俣からこの世界の様々な問題を見通す、私たちの思想を共に作っていきたいと思います。皆様の知恵と力を貸してください。そして、維持会員になっていただくことをお願いします。
また、ボランティアとしての参加、他団体との活動の連携もお待ちしています。

▶維持会員

　　年会費●1口1万円

　　特典●機関誌「ごんずい」年6回送付、特製カレンダー進呈、考証館入館無料、相思
　　　　　社宿泊無料、「ごんずいのがっこう」参加費やまち案内料割引

▶機関誌「ごんずい」の定期購読

水俣からのタイムリーなテーマを通して、水俣病事件の投げかけた意味を私たちの今の、そしてこれからの生き方・暮らし方に重ね合わせて考えていきます。バックナンバーの在庫もあります。

　　年間購読料●2,100円（年6回発行、B5変形版24頁、送料込）

▶ご寄付もよろしくお願いします

▶申し込みは郵便振替をご利用ください。

　　口座／01990-8-25341　水俣病センター相思社

①水俣病
　歴史考証館
②宿泊棟
③事務棟
④猫の墓
⑤集会棟
⑥資料室
⑦倉庫

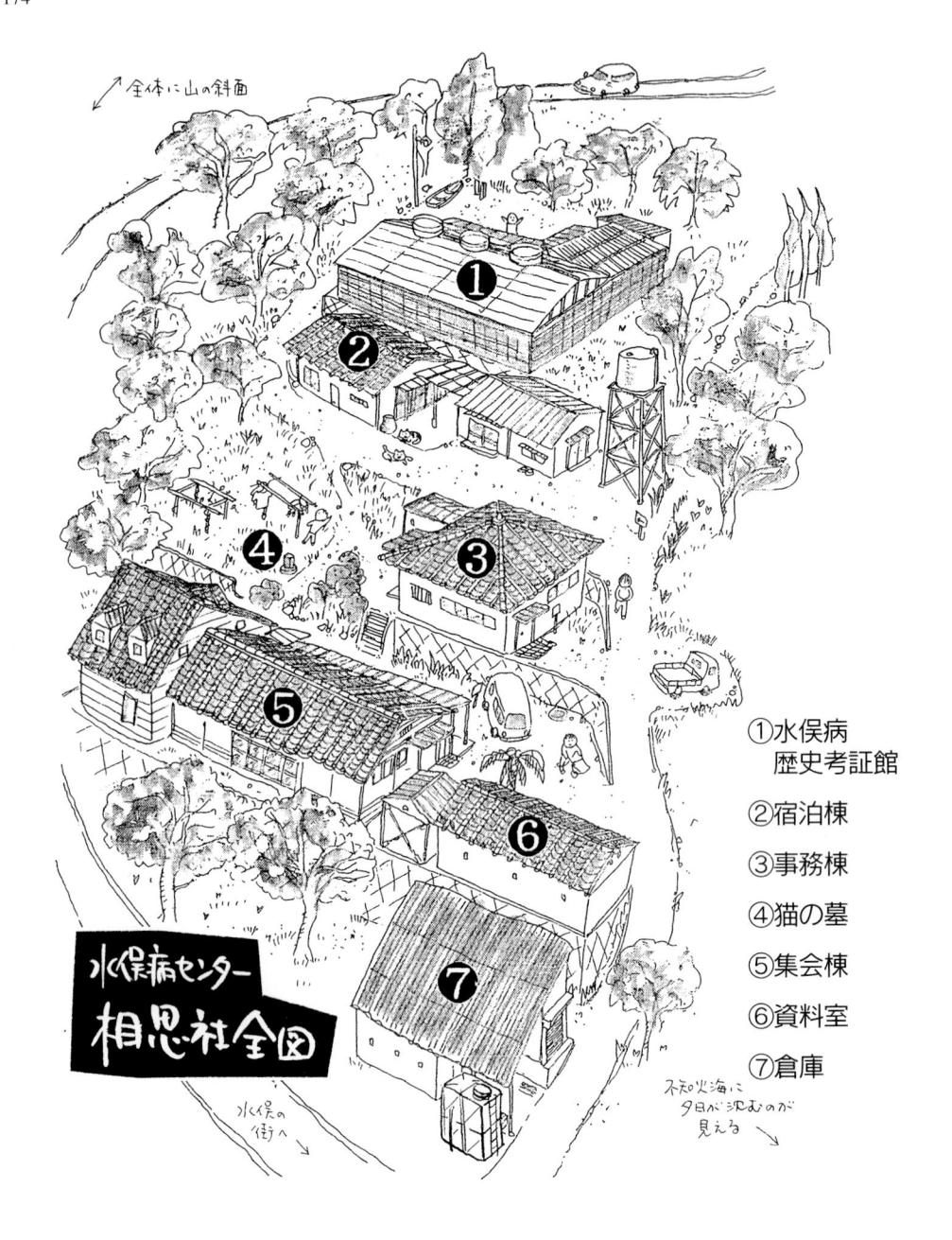

●水俣病センター相思社・水俣病歴史考証館への交通
　JR鹿児島本線・水俣駅下車
　　●バス／南国交通出水方面行きで「湯堂」下車徒歩15分
　　　　　産交バス茂道漁港行きで「月浦団地前」下車徒歩10分
　　●タクシー／約10分
　　●徒歩／約1時間

●水俣病事件略史と相思社の活動経緯 (太字)

1908年	水俣村にチッソ工場建設
1932年	水俣工場、アセトアルデヒド製造開始（水銀使用）
1956年	水俣病公式確認
1957年	水俣病患者家庭互助会結成
1959年	見舞金契約
1968年	政府、水俣病を正式に公害病と認定
1969年	水俣病訴訟（第一次訴訟）提訴
1971年	自主交渉闘争、チッソ本社前座込み
1972年	原告患者の中に「患者・家族の拠り所を作りたい」との希望が芽生える 第1回国連人間環境会議（ストックホルム）で水俣病センターの設立を呼びかける 全国から寄付を募る
1973年	水俣病第一次訴訟判決、原告勝訴
1974年	水俣病に仕切網設置 水俣病センター落成。「相思社」（互いに思い合う）と名付けられる 水俣病認定申請患者協議会結成 キノコ工場竣工。患者と共同作業開始（～1983年） 水俣湾内水銀ヘドロ、魚介類の採取と水銀分析
1975年	熊本県議杉村らの「ニセ患者発言」
1977年	未認定患者運動の拠点としての活動を開始。様々な訴訟や運動を展開 「水俣実践学校」開始（1週間ほどの夏期セミナー、水俣病の学習と交流、現在は「ごんずいのがっこう」）患者らが栽培する低農薬甘夏などの販売を始める
1978年	新次官通知。チッソ県債発行開始
1979年	「出月養生所」を設立。はり・きゅう・マッサージ治療を行う（1986年に相思社から独立）
1980年	水俣病第三次訴訟提訴
1982年	「水俣生活学校」開設（水俣病と有機農業の学習を行う1年間のフリースクール。～1992年） 関西に移住した水俣病患者が関西訴訟を提訴
1983年	資料室完成。水俣病関連資料の収集・整理・展示・貸出・資料集作成などを行う
1986年	水俣湾沿岸の生物分布調査を行う 公式確認30周年、アジア民衆環境会議開かれる
1988年	「水俣病歴史考証館」開館

1989年	甘夏事件で相思社理事総辞職
	水俣病患者連合結成
1990年	考証館移動展を各地で開催（～1994年）
	水俣湾公害防止事業（ヘドロの浚渫埋立）終了
	機関誌発行開始
	環境創造みなまた推進事業開始（～1999年）
1993年	「絵で見る水俣病」出版（日本語・英語版）
1994年	水俣の再生を考える市民の集い「そろそろもやい直しばはじめんば」の実行委員会に参加
1995年	政府、水俣病「最終」解決策を決定
1996年	公式確認40周年、水俣・東京展開かれる
1997年	水俣湾の仕切網撤去
1998年	「絵で見る水俣病」インドネシア語版・タガログ語版出版
2000年	政府、国費投入によるチッソ金融支援策を決定
2001年	水俣病関西訴訟控訴審判決
	水俣水銀国際会議参加者を対象とした講演会を開催

財団法人・水俣病センター相思社
水俣病歴史考証館
〒867-0034　熊本県水俣市袋34
TEL　0966-63-5800　FAX　0966-63-5808
ホームページ　http://www.soshisha.org／Eメール　info@soshisha.org

ILLUSTRATED MINAMATA DISEASE
絵で見る水俣病

1993年4月15日	第1刷発行Ⓒ
2004年7月1日	改訂版第1刷

編 者	㈶水俣病センター相思社
装 幀	市川事務所
発行者	伊藤晶宣
発行所	㈱世織書房
印刷所	㈱マチダ印刷
製本所	協栄製本㈱

〒240-0003 神奈川県横浜市保土ヶ谷区天王町1丁目12番地12
電話045(334)5554 振替 00250-2-18694

落丁本・乱丁本はお取替いたします　Printed in Japan ISBN4-902163-08-X

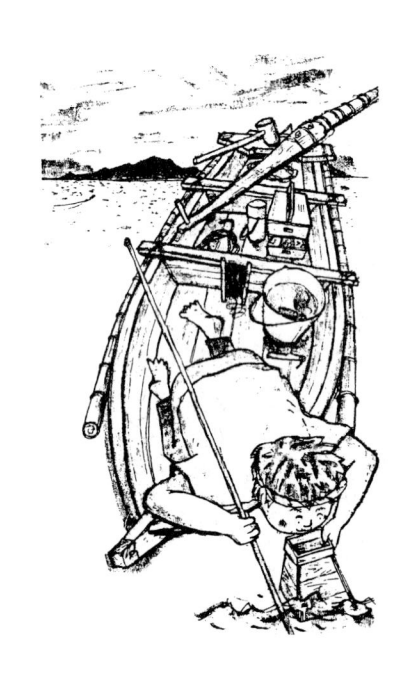

Minamata Disease Museum
水俣病歴史考証館